"The author's transparency, obvious love for the reader, and skillful guidance into unshakable hope in the midst of infertility brought me to laughter, tears, and deep soul-searching. More importantly, this book provides the reader with exactly what it promises."

DEBORAH CLENDON

"I have never read a book, except for the Bible, which demonstrates an author's deep love and concern for the reader as much as *Breathtaking Hope in the Furnace of Infertility*. To see at the close of each chapter how we, the readers, have been prayed for by June consistently underscored God's steadfast love for us and His approachability through prayer."

DIANA MAYHUGH

"If you desire intimacy with God and a lifetime of unparalleled help through your struggles, this book is a must read. Through her own failures and successes in the physical, spiritual, and emotional battles of infertility, author June Strickler transparently combines biblical truths with practical applications that can transform even the most bruised or rebellious heart into one that resonates with spiritual security and victory. Through this process, she never— for a moment—forgets the heartache of the reader who longs for motherhood."

BERYL FORNEY

"*Breathtaking Hope in the Furnace of Infertility* is so much more than a women's story of God's incredible love and hope in one of the most painful trials of life—infertility. It is a book brimming with encouraging truth of a God who desperately longs for His creation to know His redeeming love no matter your situation or current struggle. June's story powerfully proclaims—He is a God who is trustworthy and abounds in grace and mercy. That's *Breathtaking Hope!*"

GI GI HORRELL

BREATHTAKING
HOPE
IN THE FURNACE
OF INFERTILITY

—

JUNE STRICKLER

Breathtaking Hope in the Furnace of Infertility by June Strickler, published by Encouragement That Lasts, a Washington State 501(c)(3) corporation, Ephrata, WA 98823.

PO Box 462, Ephrata, WA 98823

www.encouragementhtatlasts.org

© 2021 Encouragement That Lasts

REL012130   RELIGION / Christian Living / Women's Interests

ISBN 978-0-578-71407-3 (paperback)
ISBN 978-0-578-81948-8 (ebook)

Book cover and interior design by Erik M. Peterson.

Published in the United States of America

First edition

Library of Congress Control Number 2020924907

*This book is dedicated to the woman
longing for a child brave enough
to grant me access to her innermost being.*

CONTENTS

INTRODUCTION

IT WAS A DAY LIKE many others I had experienced; a day, perhaps, like you have had. I was at the kitchen sink washing dishes and wondering, "Am I pregnant this time?" My mind and heart were as unsettled as my last meal while I battled what had become a familiar tangle of emotions: hoping we were expecting a baby, while steeling myself against impending disappointment if we weren't.

As I continued my task, I prayed for a peace of mind which proved elusive; not only did I have an absence of peace, but the very air around me began to feel oppressive. I decided I'd better start focusing on pleasant things and tried to imagine the joy we would have in a matter of days if we were to experience our first ever, positive pregnancy test. Almost immediately, however, I cringed at the strong possibility that this month—like so many others—would bring us no closer to becoming parents.

In disgust, I realized my mind had gone full circle—*again*. This "hoping to be pregnant" thing had become an emotional roller-coaster, and I was sick and tired of it. It really *shouldn't* matter whether or not I became a mother, I reasoned. My ability to live a fulfilling life shouldn't be dependent on something so far beyond my control as having children. Yet I couldn't shake the fact I was terribly wounded inside and failing to gain any meaningful victory over a grueling emotional and physical battle. The unfulfilled longing for a baby was wearing me down and turning me into a person I did *not* want to be.

Tears trickled down my face and began falling into the soapy dishwater below. *What a pitiful picture I've become*, I thought. How I hated the wondering, hoping, and pain which accompanied infertility! No matter what I tried to tell myself, I ached for a *baby!*

I dried my hands, retrieved a box of tissues, collapsed in a chair at our kitchen table, and poured out my heart—and tears—before God. For the first time in my life, I acknowledged complete brokenness. I wept in agony for myself, Brad, and the children we would perhaps never know. Sitting there in despair, I sensed the next few days would prove I was *not* pregnant and that my hopes were again going to be dashed like pottery thrown against a rock wall.

In the midst of my grieving, thoughts of my friend Dallas came to my mind. *Dallas struggles with infertility*, I thought. *She must have these kinds of days, too.* It hurt to realize the possible depth of her soul's distress.

My agony was rising, almost to a dangerous degree. I was rocking back and forth, sobbing. A memory of Emma's saddened eyes flashed before me. She was a prayer partner whose joy in life was slowly being consumed in the furnace of infertility. And suddenly, like a hammer blow, I found myself weeping unashamedly for the thousands of women I had never met who were at that moment vacuuming their floors, riding the bus, putting on their makeup, sitting at the keyboard, or trying to sleep half a world away. Women whose minds were whirling: "Will I ever have a baby? Doesn't God care? Is there something wrong with me?"

I couldn't know that God, in His grace and love, had orchestrated this moment of brokenness and grief when I would literally cry out to Him, "Lord, please let me help them! Please, *somehow*, let me help them!" My heart's desire that life-changing day was for God to allow me to encourage and help women—known and unknown to me—who were experiencing the same pain as me. The instant I made that heartfelt plea, I realized God had been patiently waiting for that specific prayer to pour out of my soul. I felt an immediate, undeniable assurance from Him that, yes, He would use me to encourage those He loved who were hurting.

As my aching mind began to revive and envision avenues in which God might permit me to do this, something unexpected happened. God interrupted my racing thoughts with the phrase "You are to write a book." I was astounded at the specificity of it, not having often experienced this type of communication from God. Nonetheless, I found myself filled with apprehension.

Why, Lord, would You want me to write a book? I wondered. I was a people person, failure prone, and far too often learned things the hard way. It would make more sense, I reasoned, for God to choose someone who was smarter and more successful to take on that task. I brought these thoughts before God as if He somehow had forgotten them. It was both miraculous—and humorous—at how quickly and thoroughly God silenced those objections by placing the following Scripture in my mind:

> But God has chosen the foolish things of the world to
> shame the wise, and God has chosen the weak things
> of the world to shame the things which are strong.
> (1 Corinthians 1:27)

Ouch! God immediately put me in my place and *then* set my heart pounding with awe. "Yes, Lord," I was forced to quietly acknowledge with fresh tears and then laughter. "I am *both* foolish and weak!" It became clear my insecurities and shortcomings were not going to be problematic to God. "I fail so often, Lord, but use me however You want to," I prayed out loud.

In His great mercy, God hid from me that day the incredible investment this endeavor would take in time, pain, trust, joy, failure, and forgiveness. I assumed the writing process would take only a few months, yet God intimately led me through it for over a two-year span of time. Those two years stretched into three, then five, seven, ten, twenty, and beyond. And while God permitted me to minister to precious friends and strangers within my peer group, He ultimately made it clear this book would contain far more wisdom and hope than I could have imagined. In His sovereign plan, it was destined to be custom-made for a younger generation facing tough and potentially terrifying times; a generation desperately in need of younger women who know and love Jesus, are grounded in truth, and able to discern God's hand in every situation before them.

Infertility (defined as the inability of a couple to achieve pregnancy after a year of "unprotected" intercourse or the inability to carry pregnancies to live birth) has plagued the human race throughout history and continues, even in an era rich in medical technology. But knowing you aren't the only couple to experience it does not dilute the pain.

Breathtaking Hope in the Furnace of Infertility provides reliable and meaningful help which encompasses your very real, physical needs as a precious soul who longs for a baby. It also honors, respects, and addresses the emotional and spiritual needs accompanying unwanted childlessness. God understands your desires. You don't want dripping sympathy or to read someone's story; you want a *baby!* And every page which follows is written in the knowledge and understanding that you long to be gently drying off your freshly bathed son or daughter and kissing the top of his or her damp, sweet smelling hair. While never losing sight of this, reliable encouragement *must* provide you with a foundation and shelter of spiritual truth and refreshment, even as it stretches and equips you for an entire lifetime.

It is my prayer that God will use the words shared in these pages to gently bind your wounds and encourage your heart; not only from the pain you're experiencing from an inability to conceive and/or safely deliver a baby, but through *every* difficulty or heartache you encounter throughout the remainder of your life. The truths presented here are tested by time and by fire. Should you embrace them, you'll find yourself in breathless awe and wonder of living life with a God who is everything He says He is.

While this book can be of tremendous encouragement to anyone in need, it's specifically tailored for the woman of God who is suffering as she prays and waits for a child. However, if you are *not* what you would consider to be "a woman of God"—or find yourself wondering what might even be meant by that phrase—this book is still for you. As you read, you'll likely discover God is not only real, but that He is neither your enemy nor unapproachable. He is holy, but also gracious and full of compassion. He is slow to anger and of great mercy. He tells us this in His Word, the Bible, and He has proven those truths to me and others countless times. My friend, God is bigger than *any* sins or failures you and I have committed or can bring to Him in repentance. *And He deeply cares about your desire to become a mother.*

I have no way of knowing where God fits into your heart or mind today, although I recognize a number of possibilities. Are you angry at God? Disappointed with Him? Not sure whether He even exists or loves you with power and perfection? If so, I humbly ask you to read the following chapters from start to finish, no matter which words, phrases, or concepts may be foreign to you (or difficult to swallow).

Perhaps you're on the other end of the spectrum and have been trusting God and walking in faithfulness, knowing He loves you and has a beautiful plan for you, yet finding yourself in need of *extra* reassurance. With gratitude and joy I am able to proclaim that God is able to meet you wherever you are at physically and spiritually right now. *You* were in God's mind the day I cried out my desire to help others who were going through the same inferno of agony I was experiencing. And even though you and I live in a world of heartache, uncertainty, and temporary fixes, the God I know is fully able to provide you with *Breathtaking Hope*. Join me, please; unwrap His gift to you in the pages to come.

1

Hope Redefined

IT HAD BEEN what I would call an ugly hot day. The furnace-like heat of the high desert sun, however, slowly gave way to a breath of coolness as night finally, refreshingly, took center stage.

The commercial kitchen I had been calling home for the last few days while cooking for a large ministry team was sparkling clean and put to bed for the night. My next appointment: Time outside under the stars.

There was an empty picnic table outdoors, a perfect spot from which to perch, feel the deepening night, and absorb the majesty around me. As I anticipated, the heavens were stunning. The Milky Way resembled a flagrant overhead river of lights in the midst of stars so vivid it seemed I should be able to touch them.

A woman whose name I couldn't recall sat down with me and together we enjoyed the glory of the Arizona night sky. It wasn't a new experience for me, having lived in the western United States all my life. But I never tired of these moments, never lost my awe of the indescribable beauty of God's handiwork (see John 1:3).

My stargazing companion finally whispered, "I've never seen *anything* like this before! I had heard about how beautiful the stars were here and seen pictures. But to be here, to experience this..." She was unable to finish.

I didn't have to look at her face to know why; like me, she had lost her breath in the midst of wonder and worship of God Almighty.

⅋

Breathtaking hope from God is like that. It isn't to just be read about or reiterated. It's personal, intimate, and meant to be experienced... by *you* (see John 4:14).

⅋

What grabbed our hearts that night under the stars was much more than the view. It was the immensity of the universe and the smallness of us, the recognition of our shortcomings before an unimaginably powerful Creator. Our understandable feelings of insignificance dissipated in the overwhelming, biblical knowledge that we were *cherished by God* (see Psalm 86:15).

The triumphant message of the Bible is that sin-stained humans have the option of entering into a free, loving, and secure relationship with the holy, all-consuming God of creation (see Romans 5:8). And it isn't us who initiates relationship or makes it come to pass. It's *God* who initiates love and relationship (see John 3:16). We're just fortunate to have the option of responding appropriately to it.

This is hope redefined: a living hope based on what *God* has done and will do (see I Peter 1:3-5). And it changes *everything*. Including life in the "ugly hot" furnace of infertility. When our culture talks about hope, it isn't anything like biblical hope, which is rooted in truth. Biblical hope isn't about the power of positive thinking. It isn't about trying to make lemonade out of lemons. It isn't comprised of meaningless pep talks or cleverly designed verbiage to jazz ourselves up.

Biblical hope is about a jaw-dropping God who knows the taste of tears (see John 11:35). It's about a God of mercy who picks us up when we've failed miserably (see I John 1:9). It's about a God who knows and understands our desires to become mothers (see Genesis 30:22). It's about the beautiful relationship we can have with God through Jesus Christ, His Son (see Romans 5:1-2). It's about truth we can count on, every minute of every day (see John 8:31b-32).

৵

Have you ever thought about the fact that the shining of the stars is *not* dependent upon our ability to view them? They're in continuous, dazzling array all around us whether we see clouds or bright sunshine overhead or even close our eyes and can't see *anything*. I find this a great reminder of the permanence of God's truths. It's God's unchanging character and truths which give us (no matter our experiences) breathtaking hope.

But today? You may be hurting so horribly that it's difficult to imagine just surviving the next week. However, there's a spot for you at the picnic table, my friend. God lovingly reserved it for you a long time ago—before you were even born.

If you choose to join me at the table and spiritually look upward, as opposed to merely reading, I'm pretty certain we'll shed a few tears together. Yet breathtaking hope begins to seep into our hearts little by little—or with shocking power—even as we wade through the nitty-gritty realities of childlessness against our will.

Through our unfulfilled longings for a baby, pain has come to call. And it has the cruelest way of ushering in feelings of loneliness which—if left unattended—are dangerous. The next chapter clearly demonstrates how this book traffics in truth. Your pain is real. And even if you're blessed to be surrounded by friends and family you might feel lonely. But like the stirring breeze carrying a trace of coolness after a hot summer day, hope birthed and sustained by truth will touch you. Because if you come to the table under the stars, you aren't going to be joining someone who doesn't know or can't remember your name. You're stepping outside to meet with the One whose power and love for you is immeasurable and cannot be described, which is okay... because He intends for you to *experience* it.

MY PRAYER FOR YOU: Father, God, I pray you will enable this young woman to find her way to the picnic table, so to speak, and allow Your hope—solid, "take it to the bank" truth—to wash over her and permeate her thinking and heart. Thank you for inviting us into intimacy with You. May we be gifted with the strength and wisdom to embrace the opportunity.

2

The Lonely Path

LITTLE DID I KNOW the experience of a teenage girl I admired during childhood would one day perfectly illustrate what many of us waiting and hoping for a child struggle with on a regular basis: a loneliness people around us may not be aware of or understand.

Her name was Merilee, and she held a key role in an outdoor play involving a large audience, numerous cast members, live animals, and significant props. Moments before she was to perform, she sustained a severe blow to the face. Anxious workers were relieved to find her conscience yet feared for her well-being and wondered who could take her place.

Unfortunately, only Merilee had practiced a critical portion of the play with her highly trained horse—one requiring significant trust and teamwork between the animal and its handler. Adding to misfortune, the play was already in full swing.

This staunch young woman convinced those around her she could still do her part. They kept her quiet and managed to stop the bleeding before she went on to perform a thrilling abduction scene, where she raced from pursuers up a steep, hillside path, dove into a deep "lake," swam to shore, and then mounted the horse without the aid of saddle or bridle. The crowd roared its approval as Merilee and her horse raced their way out of the "canyon" to freedom.

When again backstage, the support crew winced at the sight of Merilee's swelling, bruised face as she dismounted her powerful animal. A doctor was waiting to examine her, and it was confirmed her nose had been broken.

The play was a huge success, yet its heroine had been alone in her pain through it all.

Whether or not *you've* been in a performance while suffering significant pain, my guess is you can relate to my childhood idol and her ordeal.

Infertility strikes many of us by surprise, like an unexpected blow. We find ourselves grappling with pain. Despite that, "the show" must go on. People are likely depending on you for certain things. You have responsibilities that can't be ignored. You may have a few sympathizers backstage aware of your pain, yet they're helpless to remove it from you as they watch you "perform" out there.

We may have thought life would be happily ever after but instead have found elements of a lonely path.

Surrounded by people and busy with responsibilities, my heroine was very much alone in her pain that night. Surrounded by people and busy with responsibilities, you feel very much alone in your pain sometimes, don't you?

Loneliness can engulf *anyone*. Why? Because facing infertility month after month—sometimes year after year—truly *is* a lonely path. Yes, *lonely*. Even though infertility affects millions of people across the globe, the woman living with the results of infertility—including the *Christian* who has been blessed with friends and sees spiritual victories in her life—often feels alone in her struggle.

I know how much it hurts to be with a group of people when the conversation suddenly swings to their experiences during pregnancy and delivery of their babies. If this has been your experience, you probably felt as though an invisible line had suddenly been drawn, which separated you from them. You were on what I've come to call the Lonely Path.

While shopping in a busy supermarket one afternoon, I was surprised to feel a tapping on my leg. I looked down to see an adorable, brown-haired boy of about four years of age gazing off at something which had caught his attention while saying, "Mommy! Look at that!" I'm sure my eyes were wide with surprise when he turned expectantly to who he thought was his mother and received a shock of his own. "Oops! *You're* not my mom!" he said as he spotted his mother and ran to her with obvious relief. The woman, both amused and a little embarrassed, laughingly said, "Oh, don't kids do the craziest things?" She perhaps assumed I had children of my own and knew firsthand all the funny things they do to embarrass their parents.

My heart, however, was pounding furiously. I wasn't that little boy's mom. In fact, I wasn't *anybody's* mom! And just that quickly, in a crowded store, I felt isolated and in another battle that caught me completely off guard. Who would believe going to the grocery store could be so emotionally exhausting?

Perhaps you've met someone for the first time who innocently asked, "Do you have any children?" Isn't it awful to have to answer No?

Maybe you have suffered a miscarriage and, while struggling with the pain of loss, had to pack away maternity clothes you were just getting ready to wear.

You may feel lonely because not only are you childless, but you've never had a regular menstrual cycle. You may wonder in anguish what it would be like to even know on what days in your calendar year you might be fertile.

I wince to think you may have listened to other people talking about seeing an infertility specialist to aid them in their pursuit of parenthood, while you inwardly despaired because you cannot afford such treatment.

Perhaps you've tried to share your hurts and frustrations with others only to hear pat answers or, worse, been humiliated by lectures on needing to be more grateful.

Many of us have fallen prey to feeling substandard in comparison to the so-called super Christian image we imagine in others. These are individuals we see or hear about who always seem happy, look perfect, don't have dust on their shelves, and could get slugged in the mouth and genuinely say, "Well, praise the Lord!" They may be lovers of Jesus we're slightly envious of, not knowing they, too, may sometimes be suffering, shedding tears, and asking, "Why did God allow this to happen?"

Frankly, if you and I were the super Christians some of us *think* we're supposed to be, we'd never admit we feel hurt or angry, or that we're walking a path of loneliness. We wouldn't say, "It's really difficult waiting for a baby; sometimes, I don't think I can stand it another day."

As for myself, I grow sick of my Lonely Path feelings because I *know* I am a child of God who has been adopted into His family. Before we continue, however, please let me explain where the security I have as an adopted child of God comes from (because it's something *anybody* can have, and it's too fabulous *not* to share).

When I was a child, I recognized the Bible (God's Word) correctly identified me as a sinner. No, I wasn't out stealing cars (yet), but I knew the difference between right and wrong and was occasionally choosing to do what was wrong. I learned from the Bible none of us can ever be good enough to achieve God's perfect standard of purity or holiness (see Romans 3:23). These painful truths were lifted from my heart when I believed the staggering news of John 3:16, which shows that God loved us all so much He gave His only Son (Jesus Christ), so anyone who believed in Him would not have to suffer the penalty of his or her sins; rather, they would be gifted with a forever, beautiful life with God, in heaven (my paraphrase). This truth is a game-changer no matter what type of path I find myself walking. How amazing! When God looks at me (an imperfect person), He sees "June, the Forgiven and Blessed One in Christ" *not* "June, the Failure" (see Ephesians 1:5-7a). I also know He *never* leaves me or forsakes me, a promise from His Word to everyone who belongs to Him.

The Christian's confidence she will never really be alone is because God's Word is true and carries His promises that He will *never* leave her. The problem we face, however, is there is frequently a sizeable difference between what you and I may *know* and what we may *feel*. We will look at this in greater detail a little later. But for now, please don't be hard on yourself if you feel hurt or are having a difficult time with the struggles you're facing. The path we're traveling *is* a lonely path!

Yet—even though we often *feel* alone—the wonderful truth is we never *are* alone. Even if we wanted to hide from God, we couldn't. The psalmist asks: "Where can I go from Your Spirit?

Or where can I flee from Your presence?" (Psalm 139:7). Satan (who the Bible has much to tell us about) tries to convince us we are alone in our struggles. And our sinful nature, which we were each born with, buys into the lie and then we feel as if we truly are alone. Nevertheless, the truth is clearly set forth in the Bible that the child of God is *not* going to accidentally "lose" God when she needs Him! (see Matthew 28:20) And when we're feeling alone and isolated, we must stubbornly cling to God's Word. *He knows and understands our every thought and struggle!*

> O LORD, You have searched me and known me.
> You know when I sit down and when I rise up; You
> understand my thought from afar. You scrutinize my
> path and my lying down, and are intimately acquainted
> with all my ways. Even before there is a word on my
> tongue, behold, O LORD, You know it all. You have
> enclosed me behind and before, and laid Your hand
> upon me. (Psalm 139:1-5)

This passage makes it clear God did *not* abandon me that day in the grocery store when the little boy ran for his mother. Although I didn't *feel* it, He was right there with me, compassionately understanding my shock-filled pain.

I invite you to stop in your reading long enough to recall the last time you felt alone, isolated, or perhaps abandoned by God. Now picture yourself in that same situation with Jesus Christ at your side, steadying you with His hands, and whispering, "I am here. I am with you." This may seem unthinkable to us yet Psalm 139:1-5 shows God is preparing the way before us (yes, our path is custom made) *and has laid His own hand on us*. What a wonderful intimacy! The very God of creation has placed His hand on *you* as a believer. On me! We are precious and valuable to God and His love and thoughts for us cannot be measured (see Psalm 139-13-18).

Is it possible, then, what we're going through is *not* an accident or oversight on God's part, or *not* some form of punishment? Simply put: *Yes!*

King David, who wrote the above verses in Psalms under the inspiration of God's Holy Spirit, did not have my super Christian image he was trying to live up to. This man—who experienced both spiritual successes and bitter failures in his life—openly admitted God's intimate involvement in everything about him to be genuinely overwhelming: "Such knowledge is too wonderful for me. It is too high, I cannot attain unto it" (Psalm 139:6). Another way to put it is: "This is too much, too wonderful—I can't take it all in!" (Psalm 139:6, MSG).

If we skim over this truth of God's presence being with us and His own hand being lovingly upon us, we'll miss the wonderful knowledge David wrote about and become beaten and defeated (if we haven't already arrived at that point). Walking in the knowledge and belief God loves us and is with us—every step of the way—is how our Lonely Path begins to merge onto a different path: the Path of Victory.

It's easy to have misconceptions about what spiritual victory through infertility should look like, and I believe chapter 8, *What is Victory*, will work powerfully in your heart to dispel any misconceptions about it you may have. As you will see, much of what I learned from God about victory came through failure.

We won't make it to the Path of Victory, however, if we miss the important truths available to us on the Lonely Path. This

I have learned: when I find myself suffering from the pain of the Lonely Path, I need to immediately and willfully direct my thoughts to the fact that God loves me and is with me. Will you do the same?

When you feel you're on the Lonely Path, please take time to talk it over with God. Jesus said, "I will never desert you, nor will I ever forsake you" (Hebrews 13:5). God is perfectly comfortable having us say something along the lines of: "I feel lonely and hurt right now, yet I'm Your child and I believe what You said: that You are with me and will never leave me. I believe You love and care for me because You say You do. Thank You for that and please help me to face every challenge armed with this truth and have it change the way I think and act."

It's critically important for us to not only *remember* God's presence but to *allow* and to *ask* Him to help us in our day-to-day struggles. There is no need we cannot bring before God, and no subject we cannot pursue with Him. And nothing in our past or present is bigger than God's ability to help us through or forgive us for. We need no intermediary; anyone can pray to God anytime, anywhere, about anything.

The Lord is near to all who call upon Him,
to all who call upon Him in truth. (Psalm 145:18)

MY PRAYER FOR YOU: My gracious Father, You know every thought and struggle of the precious one who has just read this chapter. I pray she will recognize that You know everything about her and are ready and willing to be near to her. Help her know there isn't anywhere she can go—physically or emotionally—where You cannot help, bless, and enrich her. Give her the strength and faith necessary to call upon You with nothing held back so she can learn—or relearn— of Your care, compassion, and nearness. Lord, I ask You to enable her to trust in and experience Your indescribable presence, even when she feels she is completely alone in her pain.

3

The God
of the Lonely Path

JUST AS EXHAUSTING and fruitless as it is to try and become some unreal type of super Christian, we may be uninhibited in letting others know we are on a Lonely Path to the point it becomes our identity and a hindrance to deep, abiding joy. Things are not going the way we want, we're hurting, and we are convinced we have every right to be miserable—and we honestly find it difficult to permit anyone to work at moving us onto safer ground.

After having shared with you about the Lonely Path and God's willingness to help us when we're struggling, I'm fully aware you may not *want* to ask God to help you right now. Why? Because I know from experience that it's all too easy for us to resent the trial God is allowing us to go through. As a consequence, we can find ourselves wondering if He is *truly* all that sympathetic to help us in or through that trial.

Unlike the individual who denies the existence of God or his intervening power, the believer in Christ may be grappling with the knowledge that—while God *can* give her a safe and successful pregnancy—He *hasn't*. The God of the Bible is powerful! He is able to heal the sick, the lame, and the blind. He has proven He can raise the dead and, closer to our immediate area of concern, He brought life to the wombs of women who were beyond their child-bearing years (and even to the womb of a virgin). We may view it as unkind or unloving of God to watch us suffer the way we sometimes do when He could simply give us what we yearn for.

Hebrews 4:15 tells us we have a high priest who sympathizes with our weaknesses, "who has been tempted in all things as we are, yet without sin". We may wonder: Is Jesus' sympathy distant, or is it achingly heartfelt?

The Apostle Paul gave us the answer to that question when he recorded that Christ was "God manifest in the flesh" (1 Timothy 3:16, KJV). That is, Jesus was *both* God and man. We know His purpose in coming to earth as God and man was "that the world might be saved through Him" (John 3:17). We read that even though He took on the form of man He "committed no sin" (1 Peter 2:22). No question about it, my friend, Jesus Christ walked the Path of Victory! Yet Scripture *also* tells us Christ was "a man of sorrows and acquainted with grief" (Isaiah 53:3). What a contrast! Grief and sorrow is unquestionably Lonely Path stuff.

We don't tend to think about Jesus ever being travel-weary and in need of a shower (see John 4:6). We often fail to consider the fact Christ was homeless (see Matthew 8:20), and that it was a stigma in His culture just as it is in ours. And despite all the children's Bible story book pictures and artwork we've been exposed to about Him, the Bible records Jesus was *not* good looking! (see Isaiah 53:2). So Jesus was tired, dirty, homeless at times, and apparently even homely. These are very real samplings of Him not having an easy time of things.

Then again, perhaps you *have* spent time in God's Word and pondered what it means that Christ was "a man of sorrows, and acquainted with grief." Maybe you thought of Judas, and how he betrayed Christ. Maybe you considered Jesus' hours of agony during His last visit to the Garden of Gethsemane when His closest friends deserted Him and then His torturous, sacrificial death on the cross. Yet Christ walked this earth as *God and man* (fully human and fully God) for approximately *thirty-three years!* More than a week. Much more than a handful of months or years.

Little is revealed to us of Christ's sufferings, and even the few accounts we've been given in the Bible are only touched upon briefly. Interestingly, the shortest verse in the Bible deals with Christ's sorrow. John 11:35 reads, "Jesus wept." While this verse *is* very factual, wouldn't you agree it omits the details of Jesus' gripping thoughts, emotions, and pain?

It's comforting to know this man of sorrows who was acquainted with grief truly understands our walk along the Lonely Path. Notably, while you and I are on the Lonely Path against our will, Christ came and suffered *willingly*. We must either be amazed at Christ's unselfish love and availability to help us or erroneously think that God is love so He's supposed to love us. As crazy as it may seem, some of us have heard or read of God's marvelous love so often that we fail to regularly be in speechless awe at the magnitude of it. How do I know? Because I've been there!

Failing to love and appreciate God the Father, God the Son, and God the Holy Spirit occurs when we fail to have a biblical understanding of the horrific price He paid to free us from the eternal consequences of our sin.

Imagine having stood at a frightening location outside the city of Jerusalem called Golgotha (Place of a Skull). The sights and sounds were nauseating. It was gruesome and indescribably brutal. It was when the only Son of God, who spoke truth to the nation Israel, who performed miracles of compassion and power, who refused to succumb to the thrill of popularity, and who set His face to this precise place and time—was crucified. It was the moment when God the Father turned Himself away as His own Son, Jesus Christ, became sin for us and suffered God's wrath, paying the penalty for our sins:

> And when they had come to a place called Golgotha, which means Place of a Skull, they gave Him wine to drink mixed with gall; and after tasting it, He was unwilling to drink. And when they had crucified Him, they divided up His garments among themselves, casting lots; and sitting down, they began to keep watch over Him there. And above His head they put up the charge against Him which read 'THIS IS JESUS THE KING OF THE JEWS'. At that time two robbers were crucified with Him, one on the right and one on the left. And those passing by were hurling abuse at Him, wagging their heads, and saying, "You who destroy the

temple and rebuild it in three days, save Yourself! If
You are the Son of God, come down from the cross."
In the same way the chief priests, along with the scribes
and elders, were mocking Him and saying, "He saved
others; He cannot save Himself. He is the King of Israel;
let Him now come down from the cross and we shall
believe in Him. He trusts in God, let Him deliver Him
now, if He takes pleasure in Him; for He said, 'I am the
Son of God.'" The robbers who had been crucified with
Him were also insulting Him with the same words. Now
from the sixth hour darkness fell upon all the land until
the ninth hour. And about the ninth hour Jesus cried out
with a loud voice saying, "Eli, Eli Lama Sabachthani?"
that is, "My God, My God, why have You forsaken Me?"
(Matthew 27:33-46)

A deeper study of this passage reveals that God the Father
turned Himself away from God the Son. Imagine! Did all of
heaven tremble?

The Bible reveals that God the Father, God the Son, and God
the Holy Spirit have always been in perfect unity with each other
except for this specific snapshot of time when Christ willingly
became the unspeakable, detestable representation of sin upon
which God the Father unleashed His holy judgment. It was at
the cross of Christ where the utter holiness of heaven clashed
against everything unholy. It was here where the shed blood of
the perfect and holy Son proved to be the satisfactory offering
to appease God's judgment for not only the sins of God's followers, but the sins of the entire world (see 1 John 2:2). God's
holiness cannot have unity with sin (1 John 1:5), and it was
God the Father's role to judge it (Revelation 20:11-15). God

the Son's role was to be the once-and-for-all object of that holy outpouring of wrath at that time (Romans 6:10) and provide us the option of exchanging our sinfulness (which we tend to marginalize) for Christ's holiness (2 Corinthians 5:21). God the Holy Spirit's role was to move through the hearts of mankind, revealing to those who sought truth—and seek it today—that this was much more than just another Roman crucifixion, and what happened on that hill was no accident. He has revealed to humble souls this was not a terrible end to a dynamic leader whose luck had run out (Matthew 27:54); rather, it was a holy battle where God orchestrated the time, the place, the sacrifice, and the temporary separation *of* Himself *from* Himself... for our benefit.

The God of the Lonely Path is deep, my friend. When I remember God's promise to us that He "will not fail you or forsake you" (Deuteronomy 31:6) and "I will never desert you" nor forsake you (Hebrews 13:5), I find myself breathing with difficulty and wiping away tears. Why? *Because God has promised to do for us what He would not do for Himself!*

I became stricken with shame, awe, and worship the day God revealed to me in His Word the truth of His promise to us compared to His turning away from Christ as He suffered on the cross of Calvary on our behalf. How could God possibly love us so much?

> My Savior, My Lord. He was hanging in shame.
> He writhed, and bled, was mocked in His pain.
> The physical torture, without and within,
> Was nothing compared to the curse of my sin!

What would it be like to be sinless, as He?
Perfect and loving, holy and free.
The God of creation, of truth, and of life
Exchanging perfection for my sin and strife!

He labored for breath in earth's darkest hour
As God's judgment poured out on His Son in fierce
power.
"My God, My God!" They could hear, but not see
"Why have You forsaken Me?"

This God who gave all, turned away from His Son!
Yet together They knew the battle was won.
With a shout, "It is finished!" the Lamb of God died.
And our every sin's penalty was there crucified!

This Savior forsaken by God and by man
Knew ultimate loneliness; it was His plan.
Giving not to Himself what He's given to us:
God's presence, always, to have and to trust!

To love and to cheer us and not turn away,
To adopt us as children and lovingly say:
"I'll never leave you and never forsake!"
This astonishing promise our Savior did make.

How can I then think that You don't understand
When the pain that I feel pulls me down like quicksand?
On my Lonely Path, Lord, please help me to see
That You're always, wonderfully, ever with me!

Dearly loved one, I implore you to accept God's love and presence with you as reality:

✳ In your bedroom when your heart is breaking: *Sweetheart, I am with you.*

✳ When you are at the store purchasing menstrual pads: *I am with you.*

✳ When you wonder what it's like to hold your own healthy baby: *I am with you.*

✳ When you look at your husband and feel incomplete as a family: *I am with you, My child.*

Let us then approach the throne of grace with confidence, so that we may receive mercy and find grace to help us in our time of need. (Hebrews 4:16)

When you find yourself on the Lonely Path, remember Christ and call out to the only, true God Who created you and knows your every thought and struggle. To the God Who assures those who are His through His word:

I am with you...
I will never leave you or forsake you!

༙

MY PRAYER FOR YOU: Oh, Lord, You alone know how humbly and passionately I ask You to give this dear child a glimpse of what happened on Calvary on her behalf. Help her to see with eyes of faith that You know what true loneliness is, to have temporarily become our curse—perfectly and one time only—for our eternal welfare. Father, please help this sweet young lady to be in awe of the amazing truth that You have given to us what You refused to give to Yourself. I pray she will approach Your throne of grace with confidence and find mercy and strength to help her in her time of need. And I ask that she will call out to You and remember You are with her and will never leave her or forsake her.

4

Why Me?

"JUNE," ONE OF MY close friends in the Lord said one day. "I just don't understand why God hasn't given you and Brad a child yet. It's obviously a desire of your heart, your love for the Lord is genuine, and you would be such good parents!"

Am I terrible for having agreed with her? The Bible contains numerous passages about God's love for His children and how He derives pleasure by giving us good gifts. *So what's the hold up?* I wondered. Even though I'm woefully imperfect, the God who "knows when I sit down and when I rise up" and "understands my thought from afar" (Psalm 139) knows the true nature of my love for Him.

So, why?

With tear-filled eyes I've watched or read accounts of abandoned and neglected children. I have personally heard mothers with hatred in their voices say, "I wish my kids had never been born!" And I've wondered: *"God, if You can allow people like that to get pregnant, why single me out for possibly being someone who can't? Why? Why? Why?"*

And *that*, dear sisters, is precisely what Satan (our unrelenting enemy) wants us to do: question God and His Word.

Our first introduction to Satan takes place in the Garden of Eden, where he poses a question to Eve in a way designed to cause her to question God and His Word (see Genesis 3:1-5). That's what Satan loves to do, and he operates the same way with us as he did with Eve.

God's enemy is our enemy, but Satan—whom the Bible also calls the Great Deceiver—often masquerades as though he is a friend to us. Satan whispers that it's *God* who is working against us. On top of that, our sin nature demands we think of ourselves first and convinces us we should get everything we want (which we often erroneously translate as *need*). So let me ask: Do you ever feel as though God is dealing out greater hardship to you than is your "fair share"?

More than once, I've had such thoughts. *Why*, I reasoned, *I'm certainly no worse than her, and* she *has a baby!* Why was God withholding His blessings from me? Was He punishing me for something that, even with prayer and genuine soul-searching, I was unaware of? Or was He punishing me for something I *thought* I had been forgiven of but hadn't?

Whoa! *Stop!* When we ask "Why?" and don't have a solid answer from God's Word, Satan moves in. Let me share some examples of Satan's crippling, false answers, some tigers of falsehood he may loose at us when we don't understand why God hasn't yet given us children. We ask *Why*, and Satan nastily answers, *Because*:

> You don't deserve a baby
> God is punishing you
> God made a mistake

God doesn't really care
You don't have enough faith
You had an abortion
God isn't who the Bible says He is
You would make a rotten parent

Now that we've touched on ways in which Satan often works, is there anything you can identify as a possible falsehood *you've* been wrestling with as to why you haven't yet conceived and safely delivered a baby?

⁂

I can't help but wonder whether Satan rubs his hands in evil delight any time we wrestle with the tigers of falsehood he unleashes on us. And you and I stumble, fall, and despair over the so-called answers to our whys without knowing (or stopping to recall) that "we wrestle not against flesh and blood, but against principalities, against powers, against the rulers of the darkness of this world" (Ephesians 6:12, kjv).

The Bible shows in Ephesians 2:1-3 that all believers in Christ Jesus engage in spiritual battles from three sources: (1) our own tendencies to gravitate towards sin, (2) the pressure placed on us from the ungodly world in which we live; and (3) because of our merciless enemy, Satan (who is constantly working to chip away at truth). And, let's face it: infertility provides a strategic battleground for the spiritual warfare Satan launches at God's children. Through it, he strikes at our faith in God and His Word, our relationship with our spouse, our family, friends, coworkers, and sometimes even strangers.

All too often, we forget Satan exists, or we underestimate the cleverness of his attacks. Yet we're told to "Be of sober spirit, be on the alert. Your adversary, the devil, prowls about like a roaring lion, seeking someone to devour" (1 Peter 5:8).

I once told a brother in Christ that Satan wanted to chew us up and spit us out. I was lovingly, but quickly, corrected. Satan doesn't want to spit us out; he wants to *devour* us!

And unfortunately, *one* soft spot is all Satan needs in order to inflict serious damage. Yet infertility provides *many* soft or vulnerable spots in our lives, doesn't it? We have susceptible areas emotionally, physically, and spiritually. We must, therefore, learn to recognize the enemy and remember that spiritual warfare is being waged against us.

How can you and I stand against such a fierce opponent? First of all, we're doomed to failure any time we try to handle him alone. We must call out to our Savior God for help! Please know, however, one way in which God helps us is to teach us *how* our enemy operates.

I used the phrase *tigers of falsehood* referring to Satan's attacks on us. It's such a fitting word picture because falsehood is Satan's specialty. He *loves* to unleash falsehoods at us! So how can we recognize cleverly packaged lies that are designed to trip us up? *The best way to recognize a falsehood is to know and be saturated with the truth. Simply put, we need to spend time in God's Word.*

Perhaps you've heard the story of the apprentice who wanted to learn from the world's master how to recognize genuine jade from counterfeit jade. The master blindfolded the apprentice day after day and gave him pieces of choice jade to touch and rub in his hands and around his fingers. After many, many days the frustrated apprentice asked the master when he'd be able to take the blindfold off and start learning how to differentiate quality jade from counterfeit. The master then placed a new piece in the apprentice's hand and, upon touching it, he immediately recognized it was different than what he had been feeling for weeks. It was an imitation and not the real thing.

The apprentice had become so familiar with the real thing (truth), that he could tell when a piece wasn't right (a counterfeit). It's the same for us. We must become so deeply, intimately familiar with the truth of God's Word (the Bible) that we will be able to quickly recognize a falsehood when one runs through our mind, reaches our ears, or is flashed before our eyes.

Are you are beginning to recognize there is far more to what you and I are going through than *just* experiencing difficulties in having a baby? On the surface not yet having a baby is the issue demanding our attention. It's easy to focus on our desire for a needed nursery or admire the children of others while our own arms remain empty. Yet there is actually a *ferocious, spiritual battle* being waged in our lives, sweet friend, and infertility happens to be the ground on which it is taking place.

Satan is doing his best to knock us off our feet by tempting us to doubt God and His Word. He's slipping lies and falsehoods into our already wounded hearts. Our sovereign God, on the other hand, is allowing the encounter for a completely different reason, which we'll examine momentarily. What I urge you to be aware of now, however, is that even though we can talk about spiritual warfare and learn to recognize attacks from Satan when they come, it's still possible for us, as sinners, to sometimes get things backward and feel a twinge of bitterness or frustration toward God. On several occasions, I've caught myself wondering why God was not only allowing me to experience infertility but was also permitting Satan to unleash such ferocious attacks against me. Didn't God know how *badly* they hurt? As a Bible reader, I knew He did! So next would come that well-worn question: Well then, *why?*

Let's sit at the picnic table under the stars together and see how Scripture answers this. We're going to be encouraged!

❦

The first two truths in answering the *Why me?* question are generic to those who follow Christ and those who don't.

1. Because we are all members of the human race. We all descended from the first man, Adam (who was created in the Garden of Eden), and from him we all inherited a sinful nature. Romans 3:23 declares, "All have sinned and come short of the glory of God." One of the many reasons sin is repugnant to our holy God is because He knows the harm its consequences bring us. God created man with the ability to choose, to exercise his or her will. This free will is part of "being created in God's image" (see Genesis 1:27), which is why we aren't like programmable robots. We have exercised that will poorly and are therefore contaminated with sin. The consequences of sin are manifold: weeds, sickness, pain, unloving spouses, corrupt leaders, birth defects, murders, rebellious children, foreclosures, infertility, death, and spiritual separation from our Creator. Of course, that's just starting what could be an unbearably long and depressing list. The question *Why me?* singles us out when, in actuality, we are a part of the whole.

Why me? We are living in a world torn by the consequences of sin, just like everyone else. Unlike everyone else, however, our most noticeable struggle at this time is infertility. For another, it may be a spending problem; for someone else, a terminal illness; yet another, unemployment. Everyone on earth suffers from the sinful effects of mankind together. The believer in Christ, however, has the promise of an eternity free from the suffering of sin. Yet it's easy for us to forget this is a promise of *things to come*: "For I consider that the sufferings of this present time are not worthy to be compared with the glory that is to be revealed to us" (Romans 8:18). Wow!

Even though we're just getting started in addressing true answers to the *Why me?* question, this is the perfect time to introduce you to what I fondly call BIG Truths in a Little Box. These are truths which unlock what for many of us has been a mystery as to how this life with Christ stuff really works!

BIG Truths in a Little Box

When we recognize our sinfulness and believe in God's provision for forgiveness and acceptance by Him through His only Son, Jesus Christ, we are immediately saved from the ***penalty of sin*** (Romans 6:23). We are instantly, then, given the gift of the Holy Spirit (Ephesians 1:13) and adopted by God as His dear children (Romans 8:15) and have the promise of being with Him in heaven, forever (I John 5:13, John 3:16). What we may fail to understand right away, however, is when Christ won the victory over sin and death on the cross, He also won the victory over the ***power of sin*** in us (Romans 6:1-7). This truth has huge ramifications we will discuss in chapter 19. However, just as a baby is unaware of the wonders of how to use his mind and coordination to perform multiple functions, it's a significant process for us to apply faith to the truth that we can live free from the power of sin every day, right now (Romans 6:14). As believers, after we die physically and are with Christ in heaven (2 Corinthians 5:8), we will be saved from the very ***presence of sin*** (John 14:2-3, Romans 8:18, Revelation 21:4).

How I wish I would have understood those BIG truths while I was yet a teenager. But I thank God that I know and cling to them today, and I hope you will too.

Now on to the second *truthful* answer to the question of the day: *Why me?*

2. Because God is faithful to His creation. This second portion of generically answering the *Why me?* question may at first puzzle you. While we're all members of the fallen human race and suffering together from the effects of sin, God is mercifully showing His faithfulness to mankind by *not* letting us succeed in all problem-solving. God permits occurrences in our lives and the world which are wholly and completely out of our control. Even though the Bible states in the end of time "knowledge will increase" (Daniel 12:4), each disaster we encounter is proof that man is not in control. And while Satan and the majority of mankind do their best to tell us *God* does not exist or is not in control, God is faithfully reminding the world *on a daily basis* that He is God and we are not. None of us can say "sin isn't that big of a deal" or "we are in control" without first embracing stubbornness and deliberately choosing to live in denial of what is right smack in front of us.

A reading of Job 38-41 beautifully showcases God's wisdom and power as He directly rebukes His own suffering servant, who is unable to answer a few simple questions from Him. God's daily reminders that we are not in control paves the way for searching hearts to look beyond themselves to see God, their Creator, and hear Him when He calls. That is a *blessing!*

After recognizing the first two portions of the answer to the question *Why me?* which are generic to all people, the answer for the child of God continues on an even deeper, more personal level.

3. Because Christ desires His own to be in the world for the purposes of continuing the work of salvation (evangelism). In other words, God has not forgotten those who don't have a personal, free, and forgiven relationship with Him, and He continues to speak to the unsaved today through His Creation, His Word, and His adopted children. We see this in one of Jesus' prayers for His disciples:

> I do not ask that You take them out of the world, but to keep them from the evil one ... As You sent Me into the world, I also have sent them into the world ... I do not ask on behalf of these alone, but for those also who believe in Me through their word ... that the world may know that You sent Me, and loved them, even as You have loved Me. (John 17:15-23)

Although the above Bible passages reveal Jesus Christ wants us with Him in glory, the period of grace in which unbelieving people can call on His name for redemption (saving or forgiveness of sins) remains open. We're partly here, suffering along with the rest of humanity, in order to relate to people, sympathize and hurt with them, befriend and love them, and share with them the news of our wonderful Savior. We are here to evangelize the world; to continue the work of Christ.

4. Because we have a job to fulfill within the church body (family). Each follower of the Lord Jesus Christ should be involved in helping equip other believers to be spiritually productive. In other words, we can help others avoid or leave behind their *spiritual infertility*. Comforting others helps to strengthen and equip them. Paul tells us we are to "comfort those who are in any affliction with the comfort with which we *ourselves* are comforted by God" (2 Corinthians 1:4, emphasis added).

If you and I had no struggles or heartaches, we would never experience God's comfort, nor would we be able to be of meaningful encouragement or help to others. Comforting others should also take place outside of the church family because all people have been created by God, in His image. God has flagrantly demonstrated that every individual is priceless in value. There is no higher value the God of Creation could place on a person than to permit His own Son, Jesus, to die and pay the unimaginable price to offer that individual spiritual cleansing and a loving, intimate relationship with Him. You and I are to be genuinely caring and compassionate to *anyone* we find before us in need, whether he or she is a nonbeliever or a part of God's global church family. We'll know how to pray and lend a helping hand to others because we've suffered the pain of having our plans for children unfulfilled or slow to materialize.

5. Because we are being purified as silver and gold. Even though our suffering is *not* an indicator we're losing a battle to sin, suffering is a means by which God purifies those whom He dearly loves (see Zechariah 13:9). God is intentional about purifying and burning the dross (garbage) away from those who desire to serve Him wholeheartedly. James 1 makes it clear that trials strengthen our faith, should we be willing to let this work occur in us. James states, "Blessed is a man who perseveres under trial; for once he has been approved, he will receive the crown of life which the Lord has promised to those who love Him" (James 1:12). This purification process in us, as God's adopted children, is the same process I touched on earlier regarding sanctification (being set apart for His use) and becoming conformed (or changed) into the image of Christ.

6. Because God is pruning His fruit-bearing branches (us) to produce even more fruit. You may live in an area where there are fruit-bearing vines, such as grapes. In the land and culture through which Jesus taught, grapes used for making wine were common and even non-farmers knew the vines had to be pruned on an annual basis. Pruning was (and still is) the method of cutting out unwanted or unproductive branches as well as trimming back excellent, healthy branches so the following year's crop of fruit would be as good as—or better than—the previous year's crop. In John 15:1-2 Jesus told His followers: "I am the true vine, and My Father is the vinedresser. Every branch in Me that does not bear fruit, He takes away; and every branch that bears fruit, He prunes it so that it may bear more fruit." The fruit Christ is referring to is the spiritual fruit in our lives, a phenomenal result of trust and obedience in Christ (which we'll look at together in chapter 8). Even a strong, healthy branch will experience temporary stress when cut back for the purpose of producing a greater harvest of fruit. *Amazingly, the trusting and obedient child of God may be wondering if God is displeased with her when, in actuality, God may be doing exactly what Christ said will be done to those which are, through Him, already bearing fruit.* God personally and lovingly trims His reliable fruit-bearing branches as He joyfully looks ahead to the increase of good fruit that is to come in their lives. Just think of this! It's a bit breathtaking.

7. Because Satan attacks those who powerfully display God in their lives. We see a shocking revelation of this happening in the spiritual realm in the Old Testament book of Job. God bragged before Satan about the upright walk of His servant Job (see Job 1:6-12). And, in the New Testament we read that Satan demanded of God permission to "sift Simon Peter like wheat" (Luke 22:31). If such is ever the reason for our suffering, however, I suspect we wouldn't have an awareness of it. Any believer who is walking humbly with God would probably not, for a moment, think God was bragging on him or her! Nonetheless, we *can* observe from Scripture this is another possible reason for a believer's toughest trials. There is a spiritual dimension occurring in the heavens and on the earth *all the time* which we are largely unaware of, as Scripture fully supports. Your *Why me?* situation may be wildly applauded by the angelic hosts of God!

8. Because God is implementing His good in ways even the most trusting of His children cannot comprehend. Isaiah 55:8-9 states, "For My thoughts are not your thoughts, nor are your ways My ways," declares the Lord. For as the heavens are higher than the earth, so are My ways higher than your ways and My thoughts than Your thoughts." What does this mean? Simply and profoundly, we may never be able to reasonably derive a "suitable" answer to our *Why me?* questions because we're incapable of thinking beyond the immense separation between our reasoning ability and God's high, good, and perfect ways. This should make us feel loved and secure, rather than the opposite. God's thoughts aren't lower than our thoughts—they're higher! His workings in our lives aren't substandard paths—they are so good, high, and far above us that it reminds me of two women sitting at a picnic table on a summer night marveling at a stunningly beautiful, starry host *multiple millions* of miles above them. Even should no other answers to our *Why me?* questions exist, this one alone is all we'll ever need to infuse us with strength, joy, and rock solid hope—even in our weakest moments.

When we are faced with the *Why Me?* question and armed with one or more true answers from God's Word—as opposed to the tigers of falsehood we so often entertain—everything changes. For the better!

But what happens if we find ourselves unable to fully take all of those truths by faith? We struggle along, as I found myself doing when trying to understand how Romans 8:28, which I had known for most of my life, actually worked in the furnace of infertility:

> And we know that God causes all things to work together for good to those who love God, to those who are called according to His purpose. (Romans 8:28)

When I would try to take comfort in this verse, I found it difficult to believe God would permit a terrible struggle or tragedy to come into our lives in the name of doing something *good*. My faith was just not up to meeting the truth of this Bible verse when aligning it with childlessness. In fact, when I was most disappointed in the way I perceived God to be working, I confess Romans 8:28 seemed like a slap in the face. I was already confused with what appeared to be God's insensitivity to my pain, and for me to try and believe God was doing something wonderful through it—for *me*—was more than I was able to embrace. As a consequence, I was unexpectedly experiencing serious doubts over the trustworthiness of God's Word. And, as we discussed earlier, this is precisely where Satan hopes to see us land. If you are at that point right now, I fully understand your dilemma, even as I hope and pray for you to become free of any such doubts *today*.

※

If you were to ask me whether I expect you to stand strong in the truth of Romans 8:28 today, my answer would be, "Hopefully." As I share some of my agonizing lessons with you in the pages to come, you'll see it was a very, *very* long time before I accepted Romans 8:28 and finally clung to it with all my might. And although I don't expect you to necessarily fast-track on this wonderful biblical reality that is the believer's to claim, I know in my heart you'll benefit indescribably if you choose to take hold of it and luxuriate in it *now*, if you aren't doing so already.

❧

Yes, my friend. *Why me?* is a wonderful question once we know the *truth*. I ask that you graciously permit me to challenge you to begin thinking about a deep entwining between your very real infertility heartache and Romans 8:28.

God loves you so much. And I suspect you could use a deeper insight right now into my failures in order to understand just what an imperfect empathizer you have on your side. I invite you to turn the page and begin reading about the first obstacle I faced on my Lonely Path. As you will see, I allowed myself to become perfectly *set up* to be *chewed up* by the roaring lion!

❧

MY PRAYER FOR YOU: You are Truth, God, and I ask You to reveal Yourself and Your truth to this sweet reader who has likely been hammered by falsehoods. If she is experiencing fear or doubts, I pray You'll bind her wounds and patiently—yet relentlessly—pursue her with Your grace. I ask this

because You've done this very thing for countless others—
including me—who questioned or doubted You, only to be
refreshed by truth and raised by Your strong right hand.

5

The First Obstacle

HAVE YOU EXPERIENCED any problems of pride or guilt to deal with in regard to your infertility problem? I did, and it certainly helped Brad and I get off to a rocky start with an already sensitive issue! This problem was rooted in the fact I sometimes entertain delusions I'm self-sufficient, in control, and able to handle situations with calm efficiency. My ridiculous hope is people will look at me and think, "Wow! She's got it *together!*" I hate this tendency of mine; nonetheless, I often expend major effort to hide my faults and cover my inefficiencies.

❧

Before we were married, Brad and I agreed we didn't want any "accidents" or surprise pregnancies in our marriage. In fact, we soon decided we didn't want any children… ever. We were comfortable with the idea, even though we knew some people weren't. So unlike many women who dream of marriage and children, *I* dreamed of marriage without children. And liked it!

When people would inquire as to whether or not we had children (or wanted any), we would smile and say *No*. It was easy and straightforward. Our families were "educated," and we weren't made to feel badly about our decision. Many individuals believed we were smart—the world was getting uglier all the time and the thought of bringing children into it was somewhat frightening. They thought we had our act together and were favorably struck with our ability to deal with issues in a straightforward manner.

Our prayer regarding this monumental decision was not as strong as it could have been. More accurately, we'd both failed to fully and honestly seek God about it, doing little more than going through the motions with superficial prayer.

Although we still had no burning desire to have children, the day came when we realized we'd been remiss in earnestly laying the entire issue of children at God's feet. With this came the conviction that our lack of meaningful prayer had been sin, and we confessed it to God as such. In his mercy, God forgave us (I John 1:9).

Time rolled on. We were growing spiritually and continued to grow closer as a couple. Our life together was happy, although we were surprised to discover a beginning desire for children. We began to pray and talk about it. The desire slowly grew, and we realized God was doing a work in us. But what on earth were we to do with that messy pride? The know-it-alls were changing their minds; we wanted children!

At this point, we came up with a plan. We decided we wouldn't make a big deal about our changing thoughts for a family; we'd simply eliminate all birth control, become pregnant, and cheerfully announce to everyone the news of our baby on the way. The plans we had were great, but they failed to work out as we anticipated. It turned out I could *not* get pregnant.

As time progressed, I became increasingly frustrated and sensitive about trying to achieve pregnancy. When people would ask whether or not Brad and I were trying to have children, I would answer *No*. I didn't want them asking personal questions and discover the truth. Not surprisingly, the entire subject irritated me and I was impatient to move through this untidy little portion of our lives and get on with the next phase. In that one area of my life, I not only lied, I found myself *living* a lie!

Please let me share something. Despite my numerous faults, lying is not and never has been my normal mode of operation. Yet bringing myself to confess this repetitive sin before God was something I struggled against, for confession is meaningless without repentance (which is agreeing with God we have sinned and immediately making a complete and total change of direction). I was failing to confess this sin because I *knew* I would probably turn around and lie again the very next day should someone ask about our pursuits of parenthood. Ironically, this struggle continued only because of my foolhardy desire for others to view me as someone who had it together.

As time went on, my guilt was making me miserable. I had never been less together in my life. And although there seemed to be a still, small voice whispering for me to set things straight, I was too stubborn to do it. I didn't want to appear vulnerable. I didn't want to look like a dipstick. I didn't want anybody to say, "I told you so!"

This terrible cycle of deception imprisoned me for nearly two years. The "benefits" I gleaned from it were spiritual, emotional, and physical distress. And looking back, I realize in all probability I fooled very few people with my lying anyway.

❦

I'd always had regular menstrual cycles and assumed everything was normal with my reproductive health. It didn't help, then, when Brad took a trip to the doctor and checked out fine. This made it appear that even though I had regular cycles, the infertility problems we were experiencing were because of me. This was when Satan intensified his attacks.

Well, June, you little fool! What did you expect? First, you run along your own despicable way and do everything you can to not have a baby. Then, you tell God you're sorry and ask Him to forgive you. After that, you lie through your teeth to your friends and coworkers about not trying to get pregnant. Stupid girl! You think God's going to let you have a baby after all of that? You don't deserve one! You're a rotten Christian and a disgrace! God is punishing you. You're getting just what you deserve!

I didn't realize it at the time, but I had set myself up to be attacked by the lion—and I was miserable.

I had tried so hard to convince myself I could get away with sin in one little area of my life, yet I was paying a horrible price for that misconception. My peace had evaporated and been replaced by frustration. Guilt was an unwelcome companion, which grew stronger each day. And my awareness of my guilt was wholly appropriate: I was sinning, and it was affecting others beside me. Brad was facing his own disappointments from our inability to have a baby, and I was failing to place myself in a strategic position to be able to encourage him. It wasn't long before I was agonizing for not being the type of wife I should be and wanted to be. Of course, the guiltier and more miserable I felt about being a less than wonderful wife, the less of a joy I was to live with!

If ever a person represented a dog chasing its tail, I certainly did. And all the while Satan was whispering, *"Well, June, you little fool..."*

※

Weary from the staggering burden I was carrying, I finally arrived at the point where I knew I was going to lose my mind or have to dump the whole, rotten load of pride, guilt, and fear at God's feet. I thought of the psalmist's cry:

> Cast your burden upon the LORD, and He will sustain you; He will never allow the righteous to be shaken (Psalm. 55:22).

Righteous? Ha! Me? I thought.

As much of a pitiful joke as my "righteousness" seemed, I *did* know God viewed me as righteous because, when He sees me, He sees me through the perfect, sacrificial blood of Jesus Christ (Romans 3:19-26). As a matter of my *position* (in Christ), God counted me righteous. In *practice* (through my repetitive sinning), however, I was *far* from being righteous. As a consequence, my emotions and mind were a mess.

I was beginning to doubt whether or not I really *had* any right to claim Psalm 55:22 as a truth in my life. I knew I was a Christian and that nothing I or anyone else did has the power to "undo" that perfect work Christ accomplished in my life (John 10:28-30), but I had become so saturated with pride and lying I was beginning to think *perhaps* I might not really be one of God's children.

※

The amount of sin I had to confess to the Lord that day was overwhelming, and my faith was like a weak, fluttering candle flame. However, in faith, I *did* embrace Psalm 55:22 and cast (that is, I threw or tossed) my burdens onto the Lord. Those burdens and sins were nasty—horrible! I just threw them away from me, right at my gracious, impossible-to-understand Savior. Immediately, miraculously, I discovered—despite the fact my sin was great and my faith was small—*God took my burden away and wrapped me in peace.*

❦

I wish there were adequate words to share with you how tender God's gifts of mercy and peace were to me that day.

If you've ever been chilled to the bone by an illness and had a warm, comforting blanket wrapped around you, remember that feeling. That's similar to the peace God gave me. Praise His glorious name! When living in despair and on the edge of losing faith and heart, how tremendous I found God's miraculous outpouring of true peace! This precious passage instantly came alive, as though it were written specifically for me:

> Be anxious for nothing, but in everything by prayer and supplication with thanksgiving let your requests be made known to God. And the peace of God, which surpasses all comprehension, shall guard your hearts and your minds in Christ Jesus. (Philippians 4:6-7)

God doesn't instruct us to pray, give supplication and thanksgiving, and let our requests be made known to Him once we *feel* a certain way. He didn't say to do that once we *felt* righteous. He simply said to do it! So finally, by His compelling mercy and grace, I did.

Amazingly, God took care of the rest. He increased my faith, and the peace my tortured heart and mind received that day really *was* beyond all understanding. I felt clean and restored. Genuine joy pulsed through my being.

❦

Where are you at today? Are you staggering under a burden of guilt? Or pride? Fear or anger, perhaps? Do you find yourself wrestling with disbelief? If so, I urge you to turn it over to God this very hour. Don't mess around with any of these encumbrances like I did. It's like walking around carrying an agitated, poisonous snake in your arms. Let go and run!

Please tell God all about your struggles. He won't be shocked.

Ask Him for help. He will answer.

Thank Him for your salvation, for Christ, and the forgiveness of sin. He will accept your praise.

We know this life is filled with disappointments, and I have battled being disappointed with God at times for what He seemed to be doing, or *not* doing, in my own life. Yet when God gives us a promise, as He has in Philippians 4:6-7, He keeps it!

Think about or look back at the failures of the people God chose to have relationship with. Abraham and Jacob, for example, committed *grievous* sins. We may even say they committed some really *stupid* sins (not that any are smart). We read in the Bible about the repetitive acts of disobedience committed by the children of Israel while they wandered in the wilderness for forty years. Who was the faithful One? Not the nation Israel! It was God. Who *is* the faithful One every day? Well, it surely is not you or me. *God is!* He is our faithful, promise-keeping God, and He will never disappoint those who repent and seek the shelter of His mighty, healing wings. You and I, however, will surely stumble if we focus on God's promises without carefully considering the action required on *our* part. We're to be anxious for nothing but ask God for help in everything (Philippians 4:6-7). And *then* we will have peace. And it's easier to discover this truth for yourself than you might think. It just takes a little faith to start the process.

I love what Christ shared with His disciples here:

> Then the disciples came to Jesus privately and said, "Why could we not cast it [a demon] out?" And He said to them, "Because of the littleness of your faith; for truly I say to you, if you have faith the size of a mustard seed, you will say to this mountain, 'Move from here to there,' and it shall move; and nothing will be impossible to you. [But this kind does not go out except by prayer and fasting.]" (Matthew 17:19-21)

God is communicating that we just need a little bit of faith to obey, and we don't even have to run around trying to find it. He gives it to us! (Romans 12:3) And it's hugely encouraging to know our faith doesn't have to be impressive. *It can be as small as a mustard seed.* We just have to take one of those shaky, baby steps of faith and then let God amaze us.

My dear friend, there was a mountain of sin, fear, and unbelief in my heart. With a little bit of faith in God that enabled me to do what He said, that mountain was *moved!*

So before you continue, please take time to turn over to God any burden you may be carrying. He loves you and longs to restore your heart and mind with His wonderful, indescribable peace.

MY PRAYER FOR YOU: My merciful Savior and God, please help my friend to see any sin that may be serving as an obstacle to keep her from having intimacy with You—no matter how large and terrible it is or what we may consider to be small or insignificant. I pray she will accept Your instructions to cast her burdens on You, so she can be wrapped in Your peace—a peace so amazing she won't be able to keep silent as to Your goodness. And if she has no barrier of sin needing to be dealt with at this moment, I thank You for that and ask You to enable her to grow even deeper in her walk of love with You.

6

Waiting on the Lord, and Waiting, and Waiting . . .

TURNING TO GOD with my burden of sin and guilt was a great relief, and it felt wonderful to enjoy a harmonious relationship with Him again. I heard someone once say, "If you find you're no longer close to God, guess who moved?" I hadn't realized how much I had grown accustomed to the distance which had come between us. *God* hadn't moved away from me during my trials; *I* had moved away from Him and built a wall between us. It took a confession of sin and humble request for His forgiveness and help for those walls to come down. When they did, my fellowship and peace with God were restored, and I marveled as to why it had taken me so dreadfully long to take that faith step. Perhaps you've experienced a similar, cleansing relief and understand how I felt.

But God lovingly had some cleaning up to do, yet, on His adopted daughter, which brings to remembrance the time I salted my boss' lukewarm coffee on April Fool's day. My prank inadvertently sent the poor man running down the hallway to find a place to throw it up. I later learned that particular temperature and flavor combination had been used in his military days to make people vomit if they'd swallowed anything poisonous.

During my time of restoration with the Lord, I sorrowfully recognized I had become a "lukewarm" Christian; I hadn't been living wholeheartedly for Him. Christ shared in His stern message to the church at Laodicea just how nauseating it was for Him to be loved half-heartedly (see Revelation 3:14-22). I knew this lukewarm heart condition of mine *must* change. I found myself with a deep, sincere desire for transformation, where I would take God at His Word. I wanted to have God in the driver's seat of my heart, where He belonged, leaving me free to enjoy His strength and fellowship every single day.

With this commitment, things immediately became more peaceful and orderly in my heart and mind. Almost daily I made progress at becoming more tender and open toward God, in addition to others. My prayer life began to reach new heights (it was no longer inhibited by a wall of unconfessed sin), and I found myself turning more frequently to the Bible for encouragement and instruction. I was determined to walk by faith and not by circumstances or feelings.

Overcoming my first obstacle on the Lonely Path was a genuinely refreshing experience. And for a while, I enjoyed the equivalent of an easy walk in the sunshine. However, all too quickly, I came to realize I was *not* bee-bopping down Easy Street. The next obstacle was already looming, and for me it was very troubling. God was communicating:

"YOU MUST WAIT ON THE LORD"

Even as I marveled at how God's Holy Spirit was working in my heart and mind, my spirit sagged at the mental picture of a boulder wearing a custom-made command for me to wait upon Him! This was *not* the type of answer I had hoped for as I continued to pray and ask God to permit me to become a mom. But there it was. And the message to wait was hard to hear; as hard as the boulder I envisioned blocking my path towards parental bliss. It just *sat* there!

Silent...
Big.
IMMOVABLE.

I tried a tentative push to see if I couldn't perhaps roll it off to the side—or maybe just *squeeze* around it somehow. Unfortunately, I didn't succeed. It was becoming obvious God indeed wanted me to wait upon Him for a child. With this awareness came an honest concern that *my* idea of a sufficient wait and *God's* idea of a sufficient wait were far different. With a shudder, I thought of the biblical record of Abraham and Sarah. The length of their wait for a child was, from an earthly perspective, *horrible!* Surely God wouldn't make me wait any longer than a few more months, would He?

I was concerned that a true willingness to wait might become a test from God or a ruling to be stuck waiting *forever*. Somewhere along the line, I subconsciously adopted the notion that being *too* willing to do what God asked, or giving in to God *too* radically, would result in disaster: I would no doubt find myself living in a jungle as a missionary sharing my bed with snakes or having to eat boiled rats for dinner. I couldn't help but wonder if God's message of wait was merely His way of prepping me for a flat-out *No!* on the children issue.

Wait. What did it really mean? And just how long would I have to endure waiting?

"Lord," I pleaded. "I've already been waiting for quite a while. Can't we move on to something a little more fun? Like a positive pregnancy test?"

⁂

I mulled things over and inwardly asked: "If I genuinely become willing to really wait on the Lord for a child and communicate that willingness to God, would He then alter the path to look more like: Trusting servant. Skip the children. Proceed to life of obedient misery in Scary Jungle Location?"

How desperately I wanted to wait on the Lord! But fears and conflicting desires intervened, even though I was familiar with the words of the prophet Isaiah:

> Yet those who wait upon the LORD will gain new strength; They will mount up with wings like eagles, they will run and not get tired, they will walk and not become weary. (Isaiah 40:31)

What a beautiful promise from God's Word! It has the ring of spiritual victory about it, doesn't it? The *problem*, however, was I had *not* found myself enjoying the benefits of waiting on the Lord as specified in that passage. Far from it! This waiting business was wearing me out. Can you relate?

This brings to mind a scenario I have seen played out a number of times. An individual is waiting to be picked up by someone, and the other person is late. The fellow waiting on the sidewalk paces back and forth, back and forth. He frequently checks the time, clenches his teeth, and sighs or swears in exasperation while continuing to pace. Would you agree the man who waits like *that* is bound to go to bed *weary* at night? But it occurred to me one day I was doing pretty much the same thing as the impatient man on the sidewalk. I was walking around in tight, little circles in front of the *Wait* boulder, raising up clouds of dust, biting my nails, and muttering, "See? I'm waiting! I'm *waiting*, Lord!"

It was then I realized there are two ways in which we can wait. The first is to stew, fret, and wear oneself out. That is, going through the motions of waiting, *thinking* we're waiting, yet being bruised to the bone by it. The other is to wait on the Lord the way God was talking about in Isaiah. And just how is that? I believe it's waiting in *God's* strength instead of our own, which could be viewed as one of those frustrating, little spiritual statements that leaves most of us wondering how on earth you're supposed to accomplish it.

How *does* a person wait in God's strength? I determined to search it out. I stopped pacing in front of the *Wait* boulder, let the dust settle, and sat down with my Bible. Here is a portion of what the Holy Spirit revealed to me about *how* I was to wait on the Lord:

Dwell on excellent thoughts: Finally, brethren, whatever is true, whatever is honorable, whatever is right, whatever is pure, whatever is lovely, whatever is of good repute, if there is any excellence and if anything worthy of praise, let your mind dwell on these things. (Philippians 4:8)

Use Christ's strength: I can do all things through Him who strengthens me. (Philippians 4:13)

Rejoice: Rejoice always. (I Thessalonians 5:16)

Pray thankfully: In everything give thanks; for this is God's will for you in Christ Jesus. (I Thessalonians 5:18)

Minister to the needs of others: Above all, keep fervent in your love for one another, because love covers a multitude of sins. Be hospitable to one another without complaint. As each one has received a special gift, employ it in serving one another, as good stewards of the manifold grace of God. (I Peter 4:8-10)

These commands weren't new to me, yet I had never thought of them as a means by which to "wait on the Lord." I found myself wondering. *Why, weren't these just simple instructions on how we as Christians should be living? And weren't there many, many more to be found in God's Word? What was God trying to get through to me? That there was no complicated formula for how we're to wait upon Him? That I just needed to busy myself following His commands, to wait on Him as a servant, and keep on keeping on, as we used to sing in our church high school group years ago?*

Did waiting on the Lord involve something far more practical than kicking into spiritual neutral as I waited for a *Yes* to my prayers day after day?

The commands *Dwell on excellent thoughts... Use Christ's strength... Rejoice always... Pray thankfully... Minister to the needs of others...* drifted back to me like a soft breeze.

One of Satan's whispered lies that it's quite complicated to find out exactly what God's will for us is was demolished; God's will is *clearly* spelled out in the Bible. I found the answer I was searching for: God's plan for how to wait upon Him.

While this turned out to be a moment of enlightenment, I realized it presented me with a bit of a *problem.* God wanted me to keep throwing myself into the work of His kingdom: loving Him, serving Him, and obeying Him, *regardless of the circumstances.* Regardless of the fact I was experiencing pain and disappointment. Regardless of the fact others were getting pregnant and having darling children while we weren't. Suddenly, I found myself having to reevaluate my willingness to conform my will to God's will.

The funny thing is, I had pretty much always believed I wanted to do what God desired of me, even as I realized this was going to be far more difficult than it first appeared. The *formula* was simple: Trust and obey! But acting upon it consistently? Now that would be another matter!

Once again, I knew a heart-to-heart talk with God was long overdue. I had to tell Him that waiting for a baby was difficult, but that my desire was to willingly face whatever He required of me. I was frighteningly familiar with my weaknesses and impatience and knew the likelihood of me blowing it right from the start. I poured my heart out in prayer, asking for God's strength. Deep within, I knew He would prove faithful. Nonetheless, God clearly impressed upon me the importance of my *own* part and responsibility.

God's Word said to think on things that were lovely, pure, and good. It was *my choice* as to whether or not I was going to follow that instruction. This meant when I was on a red hot roll of self-pity, I was to deliberately force myself to stop and *immediately* begin thinking about things which were lovely. What tremendous self-discipline that would require! The same rule applied for rejoicing in Him, allowing Christ's strength to work through me, praying thankfully, and ministering to the needs of others. It appeared to be boiling down to one thing, and one thing only: *Obedience*—in all things, at all times.

Oh, no! Not *total* obedience!
Jungles, snakes, and rats are coming! I can *feel* it!

But there it was, quietly whispering to my thoughtful heart: Obedience—in all things, at all times.

౾

Just for the record, please allow me to clarify. I am *not* suggesting we can obey God's commandments and instructions on our own power. We simply can't, which is precisely what the Ten Commandments effectively proved to the human race. As believers in Christ, we need to pray without ceasing for the Holy Spirit's help for us to walk in obedience. Romans 6-8 tells us we are saved by the work Christ completed on the cross for us (a precious gift we'll unwrap together in an upcoming chapter), yet we still need the Holy Spirit to help us live out our new lives.

For now, however, it's critically important to recognize our need for obedience to God in all things, at all times, while *also* acknowledging our inability to obey God's commandments and instructions by our own power. While we cannot flawlessly obey God, *we do have the choice* every day, every hour, to either obey God's Word or to disobey God's Word (see 1 Corinthians 10:12-13). God gave this choice to Adam and Eve in the Garden of Eden, and He gives this same choice to you and me today.

If we want to experience the good gifts God has for us (such as having renewed strength, mounting up with wings as eagles, and experiencing victory), *then we must commit ourselves to lives of obedience to His Word.*

❧

Shortly after I accepted this simple truth, I had an opportunity to put it to the test. As on a number of occasions in the past, I began having pregnancy-type symptoms. They persisted. Our hopes edged higher and higher with each passing day and then our fears came true. My menstrual cycle began, and I was *heartbroken.* I had *so* hoped this time would be different! And I knew exactly how the rest of the scenario would go because it was always the same spiritually twisted pattern for me:

Step 1: Disappointment in not being pregnant/crying
Step 2: Self-pity
Step 3: Anger at myself (for being "stupid" enough to get my hopes up)
Step 4: Anger at God (for letting me down again!)
Step 5: Broken fellowship with God
Step 6: Dissatisfaction, unrest, depression

Sick of this predictable pattern and longing for victory, I found myself desperately wondering: Is it really possible for me, an average, ordinary kind of Christian, to experience renewed strength?

As I recalled the Lord speaking to me about the simple principle of obedience, I determined *this* time I had nothing to lose by at least *trying* to think right thoughts (Philippians 4:8) and praising God (I Thessalonians 5:17). Although I was extremely disappointed (which, by the way, is not a sin), I wiped my tears, told God I loved Him, communicated my hurt and disappointment, and asked Him to help me honor Him.

Soon after praying, I glanced at our old, beat-up piano. Like a sympathetic friend, it seemed to invite me to sit down and play through a few of the old hymns I had known and loved since childhood. Yet all I could do was make my way to the piano, sit down on the bench, hang my head, and cry. Before long, however, my thoughts focused on God, and I lifted my head. I moved my fingertips shakily across the keys until a series of simple chords evolved. Soon, words were accompanying those chords. A few moments later I began to sing and—just like that—a song blossomed into life.

Now we know there are gifted musicians out there who would not consider this noteworthy (pardon the pun); but for me, a poor pianist and non-songwriter, it was strange, beautiful, and wholly unexpected. And I knew it was from the Lord—just for me. He was acknowledging my hurt and soothing my pain just as surely as if He'd sat down next to me and placed His arm around my shoulders!

I'm not one to advocate "experiences" for dynamic Christian living; however, I was genuinely overwhelmed to experience God's supernatural ministering the very first time I *really* submitted myself to try things His way in this ongoing battle. Tears ran freely as words which seemed to harmonize beautifully with the melody came to me:

> Waiting on the Lord isn't easy to do
> But God said to me, "Child, it's what I ask of you."
> Help me to know
> This is another way to grow
> And help me to see
> You'll give the victory

Do Your angels wish
They could have a chance like this
To show you, Lord, they'd trust You in everything?
And can it be
You can take someone like me
And teach me to praise You continually?

When praying in His will, I sensed He said, "Be still.
This thing it shall be done; the time has not yet come."
Is mine a familiar face
At Your throne of grace?
God's timing is best
So I'll enter into His rest

And they that wait upon the Lord
Shall renew their strength
They shall mount up with wings as the eagle
They shall run and not be weary
They shall walk and not faint
Teach me; Lord teach me how to wait

Waiting on the Lord is a good thing to do

How amazing this was! I gave in to God, and He gave me a beautiful song of love and encouragement. And wouldn't you know? There wasn't a python or boiled rat in sight!

My wonder increased when, at a prayer get-together that same evening, one of the ladies there said to me, "My, June, you look *great!* Your eyes just seem sort of… well, they're full of an extra sparkle tonight."

I still wanted a baby; terribly so. But God had given me—*ordinary me*—joy on the day of my painful disappointment.

The old, terrible pattern had been broken. And it was because God is faithful, and I chose to obey Him by an act of my will. That day's pattern was:

Step 1: Disappointment in not being pregnant/crying

Step 2: Deciding to think right thoughts and focus on God

Step 3: Communicating my desire to God/asking for help

Step 4: Being quiet before God/listening to His healing words of love

Step 5: Sweet fellowship with the Lord

Step 6: Amazement/new understanding and appreciation for God

Step 7: Increased faith and trust

Step 8: Rejoicing

Perhaps you are at least a little bit like me when the hope is dashed once again, or you feel as though your dream of parenthood is slipping away. Times when you feel weak and broken. Do you continue to find yourself at the end of a pattern where you're experiencing dissatisfaction and unrest? If so, I'm compelled to ask: Where would you *prefer* to be? Riding an emotional roller coaster? Or finding yourself with a new pattern of trust and obedience where you ultimately end up *rejoicing?* To realize that you are on the Path of Victory when, by all human reasoning, you should be down for the count?

By studying God's Word and His instructions for us as to how we should live, we're on the right track to begin waiting on the Lord. And, of course, we can't stop there. We must begin *practicing* obedience in our own lives. We need to begin employing obedience as our everyday lifestyle. If you want that change, you'll find consistent obedience difficult, as have I. Consistent obedience—choosing to do right—is *not* natural for us, and therefore not easy! Obedience is one part of what I call the "victory equation." Victory is in direct proportion to our obedience to God and His Word.

In chapter 19, however, we will unlock together another truth in the victory equation which also deals with how we can claim victory in seemingly impossible situations. And once these two victory truths are accepted, your life will never be the same. I did not, however, learn the second truth of the victory equation until *after* I fell flat on my face again (in fact, more than once). Notably, these failures—enormous ones—*followed* that day of indescribable blessing God shared with me at the piano!

Before we leave *this* chapter, dear one, will you make a commitment to obey God's Word in all things, at all times, if you haven't done so already? This isn't a commitment to be perfect, but a commitment to make obedience to God your daily goal. Doing so *will* result in changed patterns in your life. In other words, you will experience your own victories.

Please don't gloss over this, because the experiences of others, such as mine described in this book, are unable to provide you with breathtaking hope. Hope and encouragement that lasts are rooted in biblical truths you choose to believe and act on. And when you do, whether you're blessed with new songs to sing or other intimacies beyond your expectations with our all-powerful God, you *will* know the exhilaration and freedom of what the Bible describes as "mounting up with wings as eagles." *Even while waiting.*

⁂

MY PRAYER FOR YOU: Compassionate God, You know how I have had to set aside fear for this dear reader as she worked her way through the last two chapters. Will she be deceived into thinking I've forgotten how much she longs for a baby? Will she think her pain through childlessness is somehow viewed as unimportant? Lord, please do not let it be so! I pray You will supernaturally infuse her with a knowledge that, as she longs for a child in her womb to be connected to her very tissues and take on the characteristics of her and her husband, You desire to have her connected and infused to You through Christ and her trusting obedience to Him. I pray she will become a mother who is known for her walk of obedience with You, and as one who flies in Your freedom like an eagle.

7

In God's Classroom

AMONG THE BLESSINGS in my life have been a number of remarkable friends. One is a disarmingly honest, lovable breath of fresh air named Paige. We met at the beauty salon; she was my efficient and engaging hair stylist, and we quickly became friends. Soon, Brad and I began to enjoy Tony and Paige's company when camping, skiing, and hanging around the dinner table. We had more and more meaningful visits about Christ, the Bible, and spiritual growth.

It didn't take this special friend long to learn about our infertility problem, and she was quick to offer sympathy, encouragement, and to regularly pray for us. The day came when young Paige confided she and Tony decided they were going to start trying to get pregnant. I was happy about their decision and immediately began to pray the Lord would bless their union and give them children quickly. And since I was working on thinking right thoughts as admonished in Philippians 4:8, I considered: "Hmm, this could be one reason why God has been holding off on our family. Maybe Paige and I will get pregnant fairly close together, and I'll have her as a special friend to share the experiences of motherhood with!" This line of thinking afforded me great pleasure.

Soon after Paige shared their intentions, I was busily preparing for a baby shower for another friend. Dallas and her husband had been signed up for adoption and just received the phone call to come and see their beautiful baby girl. As one of the members of our church family's wedding and baby shower committee, I received word we needed a baby shower for Dallas—and quickly! Despite the short notice, I was thrilled. *At last! A couple suffering with infertility had become parents!* Several of us were more than ready for *this* kind of celebration.

It was easy to organize the baby shower because many individuals volunteered to help. But our smooth planning hit a snag the morning of the event. The woman who had graciously offered the use of her beautiful, spacious home called to inform me their entire household had come down with a horrible variety of the flu.

I hung up the phone somewhat aghast. Postponing the shower wasn't feasible—the baby had just been placed in the arms of her new family. But it was the day of the shower! Where could we move it to at this late point in time?

My mind raced. We all had felt the event should be held in a home—as opposed to the church campus—for we felt a home would provide the warmest and most personal atmosphere. This meant another residence was needed *today*. On such short notice, I knew this left me with only one option: having Dallas' shower at our place.

The home God had blessed us with at the time was nice but *not* designed to handle the group of nearly forty women. However, I embraced a "can do with Christ" attitude and moved furniture, made a few trips to the church for folding chairs and began to prepare for the large group. Decorating came next. I raced to the store for balloons, crepe paper, plates, cups, ice, and other necessities, somewhat stressed at what these unplanned purchases were doing to our budget. Dealing with all the balloons, putting up the crepe paper (in what I hoped was a creative manner), and laying out the table service took up valuable time. My adrenaline was flowing about eight hundred miles per hour, and my blood pressure undoubtedly was running high too!

At last, disheveled and exhausted, I plopped down in a folding chair and examined my surroundings. The floors were gleaming, the pink and white decorations were attractive enough to look as though someone else had done them, the seating was arranged, and all necessary contacts about the change in location had been made. Everything was ready. I said a breathless prayer of thanks to God for helping me get it all organized in time. I took a deep breath and began to relax. The room seemed joyfully alive. This celebration was the result of a long-awaited answer to many, many prayers. Happiness for my dear friend and fellow sufferer through infertility engulfed me.

The loud ringing of the telephone disrupted my thoughts. I jumped up to answer.

"Hi, June. This is Paige."

This was a normal enough greeting from Paige, although something in those five little words betrayed an unusual emotion in her I was unable to pinpoint.

"Well, hello, Paige! How's it going? How are you doing?"

"I'm doing good. But, June, I have something I need to tell you." This statement was followed by a long, awkward pause.

"Paige, you're not pregnant *already*, are you?" I found myself blurting foolishly.

"Yes, I am."

I must admit I was flabbergasted. Paige was pregnant. Already? *The first month they tried?* Stunned but happy, we talked excitedly for a few minutes before she had to sign off. Paige was not insensitive in any way. She was my honest, lovable breath of fresh air.

Who gets pregnant the first month they try?

With numbness, I hung up the phone. The shock had not yet receded when I slowly turned around. My gaze was met with balloons and pink crepe paper and chairs waiting for guests. Oh, yes. How could I have forgotten? I was hosting a baby shower...

For Dallas.

And now, Paige; she must have conceived about two weeks into her quest for motherhood!

I thought of the countless baby showers I had been to for others. My memory was flooded with my own negative pregnancy tests and the disheartening timing of certain menstrual cycles.

"Why?" I burst out in frustration. It suddenly became too much to absorb. I broke down sobbing as grief, pain, and anger tore at my heart. "Why, why, *why?*" I cried as I pounded my fist on the countertop. "God, You're so cruel! To think I *trusted* You! So this is the thanks I get for caring about others? For praying for others? You answer my prayers for *them* but not the ones for myself! Why are You doing this to me when I've been trying so hard to do right?!"

Tears flowed and my bitter, angry tirade continued. It was an abyss of horrific, foolish raving. "Am I asking too much to want a baby to love and hold? It's not fair! Oh, it's so unfair! God, I don't understand You! You say you love me, but it doesn't even seem like You *care!*"

How foolishly I raved at God that day! I was wounded and bewildered. The trust I had thought as so concrete suddenly crumbled. Past victories and assurances seemed like mockeries. The beautiful song given to me earlier by God—in that very same room—now loomed as if it were a terrible, sickening joke.

The desire to pull all the shades, lock the doors, and cry myself to death overwhelmed me. I stumbled to the back of the house, fell on the bed, and wept bitterly. Time went by. When certain I could cry no more, the tears continued. But they provided no cleansing relief for my agony. With swollen eyes, sore throat, pounding head, and spiritual collapse, I was a total and complete wreck.

After what seemed years, some instinct forced me to pull myself together enough to focus on the clock. In dismay, I realized the shower was a little over an hour away—and at *my* house! Not going to the shower wasn't even an option. *The stupid thing was coming to me!*

Panic hit. There was no way on earth I could face those women that night. And sharing the thoughts from God's Word I had previously committed to do and had prepared for would be impossible!

How could I make it through the baby shower and function as a friend and hostess? How could I possibly share anything from the Bible when I had screamed and pounded my fist in anger toward God? How could I humbly challenge Dallas to diligently work to raise her daughter in a fashion honorable to Christ when *I* was the worst Christian in the world?

Was I ever in a mess!

৯৫

Just then Brad arrived home from work and found me in an alarming state. He held and comforted me as best as he could. I told him I'd lost heart and couldn't go through with the shower. Through a veil of tears, I confessed the thought of acting happy was nauseating, and that I was tired of being a good sport about being childless.

"June," Brad tenderly asked. "Do you still love God?"

What a question! With indescribable shame I recalled my bitterness and raving toward my Creator-Savior God. But even though I was hurt and confused and had sinned more horribly than anyone else in history, I knew the answer.

"Yes," I cried with a fresh flow of tears.

"Do you love Dallas?" he gently asked next.

Oh, *why* did Brad have to ask such awful, penetrating things at a time like this? I felt too exhausted and bruised to even *think*.

"You know I love Dallas," came my choking answer.

Brad took my hand. "As I see it, honey, you have only two options. You can cancel tonight's shower, or you can ask God to help you through it."

Oh, how I wanted to cancel that baby shower so I could just lie on the bed and feel sorry for myself! I needed time to nurse my wounds. But Dallas' face came to mind, and I began to realize that—as Brad knew deep down—there really *weren't* two options. Besides, I would be pushed just to get in a fast shower, change of clothes, and some basic feminine primping before the doorbell began ringing. How rotten!

My heart pounded. Could I somehow ask God to forgive me and help me get through the baby shower? And could

I—blasphemous thought—share biblical truths in a leadership capacity with the women who would be coming? When I recalled the depth of my trespass, I was appalled at the thought. How could I dare ask God to forgive me for *that?*

Nevertheless, I suddenly found I *wanted* to ask God for that and even more. I ached to be forgiven and purified, to truly enjoy the evening, and to have inner peace again—and not be a fake who was simply going through the motions. So first I prayed for forgiveness and then I prayed for a miracle of staggering proportions: to be restored and given genuine joy. Once again, my faith was pitifully small and my request larger than Mt. Everest.

⁂

How did it all turn out? Well, God did it, my friend. He performed another miracle. It was amazing to see and experience how the evening of Dallas' baby shower became one of the most beautiful nights of my life. To this day, it's a blessing etched deeply in my mind. Another miracle had been poured out on me; yet, interestingly, it came about only because God permitted it to follow on the heels of my appalling failure.

God miraculously changed me. That evening, it was as if I'd never railed at Him so bitterly; that's how complete God's forgiveness was. A wellspring of joy had filled my aching heart. And when I looked at that sweet, newborn girl, I knew only thankfulness and delight.

⁂

I was able to tell Dallas our lovable, rat-fink friend got pregnant the first month she and her husband tried, and we both laughed about it. Better yet, I was able to share it all with Paige a few days later, and we became closer than ever.

Looking back on that day, I can see how perfect God's timing was for *everything*. If I hadn't had a baby shower to host that evening, I *still* might be laying on the bed wallowing in self-pity. But God's love for me was so great that He forced the issue. He pushed me to the point where I had no choice but to quit altogether or trust Him again, so He could wash me clean and bless me with a level of inner peace that is humanly impossible to achieve. He broke me of my jealousy of mothers and moms-to-be. He brought me to a critical point where I recognized I *never* had the right to judge an individual for any sins he or she committed, no matter what those sins were, because *I* had committed the worst imaginable. I had questioned God's perfect love! I, who *knew* the price God paid for my salvation! I had been a recipient of His mercy and forgiveness over and over again.

※

Had I thought about it at the time, however, I would have had to hang my head in deepest shame and confess that, despite God's goodness and mercy toward me and the miracles He had performed, I still wasn't *entirely* convinced Romans 8:28 applied to me!

※

MY PRAYER FOR YOU: God of glory and grace, only You know how deeply waiting for a child has wounded the precious woman seeking encouragement and hope in these pages. It was for her You gave Your Son, and it was also for her, in part, You took this wretched soul and taught me of Your unfailing goodness again and again. I ask she will see Your beauty in the tapestry of her life. And when she can't see how You're working for her good, Dear Lord, I ask You to please give her the strength to be teachable in Your great and merciful classroom of life.

8

What is Victory?

WE WANT TO SEE our Lonely Paths merging onto Paths of Victory, where biblical truths dismantle cruel falsehoods at times when we're already vulnerable and hurting from the furnace of infertility. We ache for relief yet may find ourselves wondering if and when any of us can count on consistent victories and spiritual stability.

I somehow had the idea that once I experienced victory in my emotional and spiritual battles over not yet being a mom, I would then be on some type of victory track and would pretty much be able to stay on it. Can you relate?

As much as we may wish otherwise, victory is not a one-time experience. In fact, I once heard victory described as any successful struggle against an opponent or obstacle. You and I may have *many* struggles in the same battle. And our opponent, Satan, uses different attacks against us for the same old problem. For example, instead of lumping infertility into one, pitched battle, he divides it up into different, unique skirmishes. Such as your friend's baby shower you dread attending, a sale on maternity clothes you wish you needed, a painful doctor's appointment, a beautiful sex life disrupted, a negative pregnancy test, fear of adoption, the cramping pains of miscarriage, insensitive friends or family, the empty crib, and the list goes on.

It took time for me to learn the person who experiences victory may, and often does, simultaneously experience pain. This is because the Path of Victory does *not* wipe out our longings of becoming a mother, nor does it still the lips of insensitive people who may come and go through a Christ follower's life.

It's my belief Jesus not only walked the Lonely Path but *blazed* it. Yet His victories were unceasing! He remained God. He knew His mission. His purpose was fixed. His steps of obedience to His heavenly Father never faltered. The path He chose was that of victory; victory once and for all over the sin of man and curse of spiritual death. This required complete and total obedience by Jesus Christ to His heavenly Father every moment of every day. Yet our Lord was described as what? A "man of sorrows and acquainted with grief" (Isaiah 53:3). That is tough, Lonely Path stuff, isn't it?

The staggering truth is that Christ walked the Path of Victory and the Lonely Path at the same time. For Him, it was the same walkway with two distinct characteristics.

Whatever our thoughts of victory, there is no such thing as painless infertility to the woman or couple desiring to have children. Feelings of isolation and longing may continue to well up in the motherless one who looks upon the offspring of others. This is important, my friend. When you have those feelings, you are *not* failing as a woman or as a Christian. It's normal, as God Himself created us as beings with hearts and feelings. A longing for children is nothing for which to feel guilty, even though others with good intentions may try to tell us differently. We must face the facts. Some things in life just cause pain. And infertility when we desire children is one of them.

We *can* experience pain and feelings of loneliness without wallowing in sin. Just as it isn't sin to be tempted, it isn't sin to have human experiences. As with temptation, however, it's our *response* to it that can become sin.

From the previous chapter, you were able to see the unfolding of a human experience which became sin as I reacted to my feelings of isolation in the wrong manner. Again, my desire to become pregnant and have a baby wasn't wrong, but my explosive anger at God for His timing and His ways *was* wrong. Terribly so!

All this to say, please don't look down on yourself, or anyone else, who doesn't yet appear to have had a merging of her Lonely Path with the Path of Victory. The one struggling along may be doing so without sinning.

As I shared earlier, victory—in part—is in direct proportion to our obedience to God and His Word. Because of this, victory is *not* something every believer will automatically experience, even over time. Being a Christian doesn't guarantee that a woman undergoing infertility will find her Lonely Path merging onto the Path of Victory. God allows each of us to make that individual choice.

Since there will still be pain, disappointment, and attacks from Satan while we're on the Path of Victory, we may ask what the difference is between it and the Lonely Path? Amazingly, the Path of Victory is easier to navigate and, at the same time, much, much harder. The Bible addresses how our eternal destiny choices also have applicability to our daily walk:

Enter by the narrow gate; for the gate is wide and the way is broad that leads to destruction, and many are those who enter by it. For the gate is small and the way is narrow that leads to life, and few are those who find it. (Matt. 7:13-14)

The majority of mankind cruises on a wide, paved highway of spiritual falsehoods and misconceptions, ranging all the way from disbelief in God to believing and exalting unbiblical teachings about God. The Bible indicates this is easy for us to do because of our inherent sin nature. However, from the mouth of Christ comes clear teaching about the narrow gate and the narrow pathway—one that isn't possible to smoothly cruise on.

There *is* a narrow pathway to life. Yet the world around us is working tirelessly to maintain the broad highway to destruction. There are limitless road crews and equipment going at it full time, and different individuals recognize (or give honor to) different road crews. They work under the banners of self-sufficiency, philosophy, self-realization, sophistication, or religion, to name just a few. The world says traveling any other road than the broad highway is stupid or weak.

My friend, it's far easier for us to rage, fume, and become embittered through infertility (or any other trial) than it is for us to focus on God and yield ourselves through obedience and submission to Him and His Word. The reason the Path of Victory is more difficult to walk is because it is in direct opposition to the beliefs and standards of the society in which we live and the purposes of Satan, who Jesus identified as the "ruler of this world" (John 14:30). On more than one occasion Christ warned those who seemed eager to follow Him to think it over carefully. He made it clear it would be difficult, and they should first count the cost (Luke 14:28).

From this, we can only conclude the cost is potentially great. Jesus was very clear about the way to life in Him being through death to our self will. He said we should take up our cross and follow Him (Matthew 16:24) and that we should expect hatred from the world (John 15:19).

It took no time at all for Christ's followers to see the truth of His teachings. Most of the twelve disciples were martyred for their faith and multiple thousands of followers of the Lord Jesus Christ have died for their faith since then. Christian men, women, teenagers, and children are being persecuted and/or martyred while you're working your way through this book. Jesus *never* presented an "easy believe-ism" platform to His listeners.

Walking the Path of Victory is walking in obedience to the God of creation. It's tough! It means moving out of our comfort zones. And when we take steps to move out of our comfort zones, we're *not* the only ones who become uncomfortable. Christians and non-Christians alike may begin to call us a variety of disturbing names. The obedient Christian walk is not for spineless wimps. It's going upstream in a downstream world. It means making a conscientious act to kill natural thoughts and desires that are wrong (Colossians 3:5).

It's possible when choosing the less traveled route that we may go from enjoying a certain amount of regard from others to suddenly becoming outcasts of our own society. And Satan isn't asleep at the wheel when it comes to opposing God's beloved children. He's quick to employ our own sin nature and the society he controls, most often without that society's awareness, to attack us with renewed zeal.

I was literally attacked by some red ants one day. Those things were *nasty!* But I noticed something interesting about them. They didn't find a way to race into the house and seek me out. I did *not* see an army of them coming straight at me with vicious intent written all over their little red faces while I was indoors. But when I unknowingly got on *their* home turf when trimming the lawn, the next thing I knew, there they were and the attack was on!

When we're on the Path of Victory, sweet friend, we're actually stepping on Satan's toes. *We are messing up his turf.* Suddenly, we've become a threat to him. Like the ants, this stirs him up for battle quicker than anything.

Satan doesn't *want* society to see one of Christ's followers walking in victory and obedience. His stranglehold on society would be weakened by the impact of such a remarkable life.

If you're beginning to wonder whether victory is worth the struggle, please bear with me a little bit longer. Just as the spiritual battles are most often greater on the Path of Victory, the spiritual blessings are *incomparably* so!

It took me a long time to really appreciate what a blessing the fruit of the Spirit is as outlined in Galatians 5:22-23. This fruit cannot be purchased at our local grocery stores; neither can we obtain it by buying a certain book or download, through attending a wonderful seminar, or even by being with the "right" friends or church family. There is only *one way* to come into the possession of it. These characteristics of God's Holy Spirit take root and bloom only in the heart that is under God's control; namely, the heart of an obedient follower of Jesus Christ.

Even though this fruit is exhibited in the characteristics listed below, it's *a* fruit, a package deal so to speak. If we fail to exhibit all the characteristics of the fruit of the Spirit at any given time, it simply means not all areas of our life are under God's control.

The fruit of the Spirit is love, joy, peace, patience, kindness, goodness, faithfulness, gentleness, and self-control. When we walk the Path of Victory (that is, obedience and submission to God), this fruit will characterize our lives.

> And the one who keeps His commandments abides in Him, and He in him. And we know that He abides in us, by the Spirit whom He has given us. (1 John 3:24)

How do we recognize the Holy Spirit? By the fruit. If, as Christians, we're failing to see that fruit consistently in our lives, we can know it's because we are failing to keep God's commandments and are not truly abiding in Him. When the believer remains under the control of the Holy Spirit in the midst of conflict, the fruit will still be present and operating— even in times of great pain.

It's this refreshing, incredible fruit which makes walking on that narrow pathway easier. The Path of Victory *does* have war-fare, pain, and conflict, yet the taste of the fruit of the Spirit not only builds the believer up but affords him or her blessings which well up in the heart and before long bubble out in words of praise and thanksgiving to God. The psalmist declares: ""O taste and see that the Lord is good; How blessed is the man who takes refuge in Him!" Psalm 34:8.

❧

So now I must ask: What price would you be willing to pay today for peace through infertility? Aren't you like me? *I need that fruit!* How I need to be love-inspired, love-mastered, love-driven and to exhibit joy and self-control. The fruit of the Spirit is the victory banquet in the obedient Christian's life.

Committing to walk the Path of Victory and obedience is much like committing to a tough, sweaty hike—complete with leg cramps and protesting lungs. Yet the views to behold, the scenery along the way, and the breathtaking vistas of God's mighty hand make that narrow, more difficult path a privilege to walk.

We *immediately* get off the victory trail any time we choose to do things our way instead of God's way. So it's true we can experience victory one moment yet feel it slipping through our fingers another. Until we see Christ and are made perfect in His image (I John 3:2), we will have trouble staying on the victorious path. Knowing this in advance, however, we can watch for pitfalls, dust ourselves off (with God's gracious help) after a fall, and walk in obedience and victory again. And, really, obedience is like anything else. The more we practice it, the better we'll get at it.

God is *pleased beyond measure* to help us in this area. Unlike the well-intentioned person without Jesus who tries to live a good and moral life, the Christ follower has God's Spirit to draw from as he or she endeavors to do His will. As you practice obedience, you will begin to see more consistent victories, and they will bless you mightily. The time will then come when you've slipped into sin and you quickly recognize the absence of the fruit of the Spirit in your life. You'll find yourself wanting to get back on the right track right away because you will know almost instantly what it is that you're missing: *victory.*

❦

This chapter addresses *our* part in the victory equation—obedience. And it will be a full-time job for you to seek after God with an obedient heart in all things at all times, as I am challenging you to do. Little did I know, however, God would one day lead me to an Olympic museum halfway across the world to provide us with a most remarkable example to the second part of the victory equation.

This chapter may seem overwhelming with the amount of commitment and hard work that is due on our part. Be that as it may, when we come to understand what *God's* part was (and is) in our victory equation, we won't help but be filled with joy and gratitude. Like me, you may audibly lift up in worship a very holy *Hallelujah!*

Move over, Lonely Path. Victory is available for this dear reader, as proven through this failure-prone author!

MY PRAYER FOR YOU: Thank You, Lord, for loving us so deeply and for the way You've shown us Your heart through Your Son and Your Word. Please cause this dear child to long for spiritual victory. May she pursue You and spiritual excellence through her will and the power of Your Holy Spirit. I ask You to give her the strength to trust in You at a greater level than she ever has, and that You'll permit us to be shoulder to shoulder in heaven one day, shouting and singing with one heart of how You delivered us from ourselves, the enticements of this world, and our enemy of old. Lord, enable her to taste and see that You are good!

9

The Worthy Goal

WAITING ON THE LORD, learning to recognize spiritual battles, believing God's Word to be 100 percent true all the time, and growing in faith and obedience do *not* happen in a 1-2-3-step process. Nonetheless, one area is much like the glue which holds quite a bit of it together—and it has to do with *you*.

What is your goal in life? Do you have a *life* goal?

You may wonder how having a worthy goal could have anything to do with coming into the possession of needed, breathtaking hope. I'm fighting tears for you as I write because I know you ache to have a child of your own to love and hold, and I cannot give you that. What I *am* able to do through God's grace, however, is invite you to wrestle with me and God's Holy Spirit through some critical questions. If you'll permit this to occur, I know you will be blessed, and that blessing will shine onto others and have an impact for generations to come. If we were sitting at the picnic table together, I'd reach out, gently squeeze your hand, and humbly ask of you the following questions:

Is your goal in life to be a good wife?

Is it to become financially secure?

To become the vice president of the company you work for?

To be the best housekeeper around?

Is your goal in life to become a mother?

There is nothing wrong with setting goals for oneself. In fact, as a married woman there would be something drastically wrong with me if being an excellent wife wasn't one of my goals. Yet what if it was my life goal and Brad died next week?

This is actually kind of scary. If we don't have a worthy life goal, we'll end up with goals and aspirations that are precariously dependent on multitudes of circumstances. When this happens, it's difficult for us to determine what we're really doing with our life or what is even most important to us. It leaves the door wide open for disappointment, frustration, or mediocrity. Goals relating to our family, finances, physical health, and such are essential. More important, however, is my ultimate goal or objective. What is yours?

꙳

Just as some of our goals may be frustrated by events beyond our control, some of us have goals we may be able to achieve. Perhaps it's a dream house or car we desire. Personally, I would *love* to have a mint condition white 1965 Corvette with blue interior and factory air-conditioning. My love for this particular car has been with me for years.

One day, I was driving home from work and actually *saw* my dream car parked at a business with a *For Sale* sign in the window. I turned into the parking lot and was practically drooling even before getting out of my boring vehicle. As one half of a couple who was hoping to have children and needed to be saving every dime possible (and—oh yeah—should have a vehicle with room for car seats), it was pretty silly of me to be standing in a parking lot looking at a Corvette like some starry-eyed, teenaged boy!

More important than succeeding in some of our goals about where we live or what we drive, some of us may have our dream or goal to become a mother realized. Yet while God often allows us extras over and above our needs, He's more concerned with what thoughts we harbored in our minds today than how we got from point A to point B, or even whether or not we were playing with a very lovable son or daughter.

When we see Christ face-to-face, we will *not* be giving any thoughts to vehicles we enjoyed, what our home looked like, or even whether our desire to become a mom was fulfilled. Suddenly, what's going to matter most to each and every one of us is that we lived a life of faithfulness to God, we strove to become more Christ-like, and we saw things with spiritual eyes.

The Apostle Paul was able to say of himself, "I have fought a good fight, I have finished my course, I have kept the faith" (2 Timothy 4:7). Paul didn't have to ponder what his goal in life was. Out of gratitude for what Jesus Christ had done for him, and out of an understanding of the breathtaking hope God provides His children for the present *and* the future, Paul wanted to give his all for Jesus Christ. That passion was constantly before him, and keeping it was his number one priority.

Paul's personal needs and natural desires weren't swept away, but they were of secondary importance to him. He had learned to become flexible about his needs and desires and inflexible regarding his worthy life goal.

Seeing Christ face-to-face is a coming reality I tend to forget. When there are meals to cook, appointments to be made, friends getting pregnant, and all kinds of ordinary occurrences constantly before me, the idea of living in Christ's presence is often relegated back to some fuzzy, cobwebbed recess of my mind.

Everyday living with its routines and responsibilities just happens to be a normal part of life. Despite this fact, I need to focus daily that this world is *not my home*. As a child of God, my real home and citizenship is in heaven (see Ephesians 2:19). I need to discipline myself to think of what it is God wants to use me for on this earth today as His beloved child.

Perhaps this is a discipline you need as well. Our earthly days are numbered! What are we doing with the fleeting hours, days, and years which holds importance not only to us but for God's kingdom?

As a dear friend of ours challenged me about my goal in life, I began to realize the proper life goal would not separate everyday living from worthy spiritual pursuits. In fact, I've come to learn that everyday living is the *playfield* for our spiritual exercises and encounters.

❧

"I have fought a good fight, I have finished my course, I have kept the faith" (2 Timothy 4:7). What a wonderful thing this would be for *each* follower of the Lord Jesus Christ to be able to say at the end of his or her life! So why could Paul make those statements? It was because his goal was to model Christ to the best of his ability, and he strove to model Him a day at a time, an hour at a time. Through this process, however, Paul kept what I will call a "sane estimation" of himself (see Romans

12:3). He didn't delude himself or try to convince others into thinking that he "had it all together" (as I tried in vain to do). Paul remembered his own tendencies to sin and was fully cognizant of his weaknesses and inability to do anything worthwhile through his own power (see Romans 7:15).

This excites me, my friend. Why? Because *God will joyfully fellowship with and use any person like that!* When you and I have a life goal in keeping with God's Word and recognize the fact *God alone* can help us in this goal, we'll be humble and running on course.

With encouragement and insight from a Godly couple, I've been blessed to embrace a life goal which isn't conditioned by *any* circumstance or situation facing me. That goal is to become like Christ. This means being continually controlled by the Holy Spirit, which, of course, is another way of saying that I'm committing myself to being obedient to God and His Word without any exceptions.

Whew! Will I succeed? I can hope so, even as I recognize there will be multiple failures—often by the hour. However, I have come to learn I shouldn't stress about failing. A goal is something we reach for, something which causes us to stretch. Christ-likeness is the highest goal I see the Bible exhorting us to embrace. It is an indescribably high goal, but *it will be a lifelong endeavor for me.*

It's amazing that mere mortals can even discuss or consider becoming *anything* like Christ; only a gracious, all powerful God can offer us that impossible option.

God greatly encourages me in my life goal through the writing of Paul:

Brethren, I do not regard myself as having laid hold of it yet; but one thing I do: forgetting what lies behind and reaching forward to what lies ahead. I press on toward the goal for the prize of the upward call of God in Christ Jesus. (Philippians 3:13-14)

Another passage of loving exhortation for this journey is found in Romans:

I urge you therefore, brethren, by the mercies of God, to present your bodies a living and holy sacrifice, acceptable to God, which is your spiritual service of worship. And do not be conformed to this world, but be transformed by the renewing of your mind, that you may prove what the will of God is, that which is good and acceptable and perfect. (Romans 12:1-2)

My goal, to be like Christ:

For through the grace given to me I say to every man among you not to think more highly of himself than he ought to think; but to think so as to have sound judgment. (Romans 12:3).

You see, I'm under no illusions as to my shortcomings. I'm not some type of super Christian because I've zeroed in on a worthy life goal. If you lived with me, you'd see me struggle with anger and rotten attitudes toward others, for my sin nature is ever fighting for control. And all too frequently, I seem almost *eager* to cave into temptation (to my later disgust). Yet what I do have now, even though I often fail at it, is a clear, easily defined goal or purpose in my life. It interrupts my thought life. It changes my priorities. And, unlike many other worth-while goals, my ultimate goal—to become like Christ—*is not dependent upon or affected by any circumstances:*

* Even should my husband die next week.
* Whether our country is at peace or at war.
* Whether I'm healthy or paralyzed.
* Whether or not God allows me to have children.

Is hoping to have a child still extremely important? *Absolutely!* The desire for children is beautiful and precious. And please bear in mind that if you readjust your ultimate goal in life—which you may need to do—other goals, such as improving your relationship to your husband, better managing your money, and taking steps to become a parent are still very worthwhile and necessary.

※

I love the heart behind the below, old hymn:

I'd rather have Jesus than silver or gold;
I'd rather be His than have riches untold;
I'd rather have Jesus than houses or lands.
Yes, I'd rather be led by His nail-pierced hands.

Than to be the king of a vast domain
and be held in sin's dread sway.
I'd rather have Jesus than anything
this world affords today.

I'd rather have Jesus than *anything*. Is that true in my heart? It is at this moment, and I pray fearfully God will keep it so. Would I *really* rather have Jesus than comfort, my husband, or having children? It's a question I should ask myself in the quiet of each day.

How about you?

Do you have a life goal? If so, is it a worthy goal in view of eternity? What is going to matter most when you see Christ face-to-face?

❧

Neither God or I have suddenly turned insensitive about your intense, understandable longing for children, and I trust you know that. Nevertheless, these questions about your goal in life are unavoidable if there is to be breathtaking healing and purpose through your struggle. *And that is my primary concern.* It would be thrilling for me to learn you have adopted or given birth to a baby! Yet in all honesty, I would be just as thrilled—undoubtedly more so—to learn your focus goes beyond this life with its dreams and cares, however worthwhile, and rests on Christ the solid Rock.

Oh, I hope you *do* become a mother! A mother who, *by her life*, imparts to her children what is *truly* most important.

❧

MY PRAYER FOR YOU: Holy Father, I humbly ask You will enable this dear child to grasp what is most important today, tomorrow, and for the remainder of her life. May Your Holy Spirit guide her thinking as she takes stock of her priorities. Please encourage her in Your patient and wonderful way, bringing her to a freeing abandonment of any fear of trusting You wholeheartedly in every aspect of her life. In tears I plead: Let her become a woman of great spiritual truth and influence into the next generation, and into many others to follow.

10

Gagging on Flour

EVEN AS I FOCUSED on my goal and desire to be like the Lord Jesus, I felt as if God were making me gag on a bowl of flour. I know this sounds bad, but it's the truth. And it had to do with my continuing battle over the Bible verse you've heard so much from me: *"And we know that God causes all things to work together for good to those who love God, to those who are called according to His purpose"* (Romans 8:28).

God was working to show me the deep meaning of this portion of His Word. He just wouldn't let go of the fact He was acting in love and mercy in my life, even as I struggled and wept my way through myriads of hurts and fears relating to infertility.

"All things work together for good." *God, please don't be displeased with me,* I inwardly plead. *I know Your Word is true! But it is such a tough faith issue to see how not being a mom can be good. It's awful, Lord! Teach me!*

God was unbelievably patient. The Holy Spirit whispered for me to slow down and read this Bible verse in context. Only after doing so did I see that Romans 8:28 does *not* state "all things are good." I had sort of been reading it that way and gagging on it. Rather, this verse states "God causes all things to *work together* for good."

Oh! I thought. *That does change things a bit.* And it made me think of... well, baking a cake.

This is especially humorous as Brad did *not* start married life with a wife who was a good cook. My interests had previously been in outdoor activities, and I knew more about how a tennis racket should be strung than how to cook a roast. Nonetheless, I *did* know more than to set a bowl of flour in front of my man, sweetly smile, and announce I had made him a cake. Oh, certainly one of the *ingredients* in my husband's favorite cake was flour, but flour alone wasn't enough. *Disgusting!*

If I may put it this way, our infertility is not unlike flour. All by itself, it really *is* awful. But God is making something good, both for us and His kingdom, and the "flour" (infertility) will be used in conjunction with other things to make something unimaginably good. Like a master chef, God has been graciously and carefully placing ingredients in our lives, my sister-friend. It means our pain is not wasted or random. This is *precisely* what is happening *if* we are individuals who are described by the second half of that verse: "all things work together for good to them that love God, to them that are called according to His purpose."

Have you ever caught the fact this thrilling truth is null and void for anyone who does not (a) *love* God or (b) is not *called according to His purpose?*

Hmm, we should subsequently be asking ourselves: How can I tell if I truly love God or simply *think* I love God?

The Lord Jesus explains: "If you love Me, you will keep My commandments" (John 14:15). Later in the chapter Jesus is equally clear: "He who has My commandments and keeps them is the one who loves Me" (John 14:21).

Do you, precious one, fit the first qualifier listed in Romans 8:28? Do you love God? Your obedience to Him—even through the tough battles and disappointments of infertility—is a measuring rod for determining your heart's true love condition toward Him. Suddenly, it's uncomfortably easy to pinpoint exactly where we are.

> And by this we know that we have come to know Him,
> if we keep His commandments. The one who says,
> "I have come to know Him" and does not keep His
> commandments, is a liar, and the truth is not in him.
> (1 John 2:3-4)

These passages, of course, aren't saying if an individual *ever* fails to keep God's commandments and instructions, he or she does not love God or isn't His child. Rather, it's directing our attention to a pattern in an individual's life; a habit, a lifestyle. Is it your habit or goal to believe and obey God's Word regardless of the circumstances in which you find yourself?

Look at the last portion of Romans 8:28: "to them that are called according to His purpose." Unfortunately, this is a neglected teaching, and you may be wondering what it means. Let's look at it this way. When younger, do you remember being called to supper? Supper was ready, and you were invited or called to come and take part in that meal.

In a similar way God calls those who become His children. Through the Bible and the Holy Spirit we learn about our sin nature and God's redemptive plan of salvation for those who place their faith and trust in His Son, Jesus Christ. We are *invited* or *called* to partake in eternal life in Christ. Yet there is far more to it than that. We are called according to *His* purpose.

This means we aren't adding Christ to our life to "round it out" or make sure we "go to heaven" after we physically die. Being called according to His purpose is recognizing and believing He did all the work necessary for our salvation which—when properly understood—should result in us laying our very lives at the feet of the Savior and saying, "Use me however you want; I'm making you Lord and Master of my life." It means answering the call to do things God's way instead of our own. It means His desires become our desires and His plans become our plans.

To be "called according to His purpose" means to respond to God's call and loving pursuit of us with a willingness to do what He wants us to do and be what He wants us to be, regardless of what we see going on—or failing to happen—in our lives.

The question each of us should probably be asking is this: Is God in my life to attend to my needs and desires or is God my life?

When we become willing to answer God's call of committing ourselves to His purposes, we can then herald the wonderful promise of Romans 8:28. We then have additional assurances in black and white that the trials we undergo are *not* meaningless. Our faith should be able to rest in the knowledge that God has a purpose for what we are going through, and in His Word we're told it is a *good* purpose. Now *this* gets exciting!

God used the word *good* at the start of His written communication to mankind. It's a descriptive word for the work God had done in creating the sun, moon, and stars, and the earth with its grass, trees, and beautiful variety of flowering plants and food. It's the same word He used to describe the animals He created and placed on the land and in the sea, and the same word He used to describe His creation of mankind. Read Genesis 1. Over and over the phrase "and God saw that it was good" is used.

Good? It seems as if God understates the fabulous!

Have you ever seen a rugged mountain range in the fall when the peaks are wearing a fresh mantle of snow with the bluest sky imaginable as a backdrop? Have you ever felt the spray from a thundering waterfall, watched a horse run free, or seen a brightly colored flower growing through a crack in a rock? Have you observed a storm moving over the desert or a bird soaring effortlessly hundreds of feet up in the air? What God described as good has, on occasion, rendered me speechless because I knew of no words to adequately describe the beauty of His creation.

This same God is telling you and me today that "God causes all things to work together for good to them that love God, to them that are called according to His purpose."

Can infertility really be working with something else to bring about good in our lives? Good in *God's* definition of the word? My tears flow at the thought. Only this time they're tears of wonder and awe. How little I have known God!

Does this make childlessness against our will an easy experience? *No!* The pain and the struggles we face are real and very,

very difficult. Infertility will *never* be easy for you and me to live with. But remember: God understands that, and He cares. And for the child of God who is called according to His plans, *it has a good and worthwhile purpose.* James tells us one aspect of that purpose, and it really is staggering:

> Consider it all joy, my brethren, when you encounter various trials, knowing that the testing of your faith produces endurance. And let endurance have its perfect result, that you may be perfect and complete, lacking in nothing. (James 1:2-4)

Believe it or not, more of that purpose was shown to me in the most awful, remarkable way through some spilled spaghetti sauce, which really ticked me off. And, as you will soon see, it was all over a fierce, horrific battle I took up against God over… you guessed it, *Romans 8:28.*

ॐ

If you aren't buying into Romans 8:28 yet, please do *not* lose heart! You're not beyond help or the ability of receiving breathtaking hope in this furnace of infertility. And God has spared my life in more ways than one so I can share this with you, my friend!

ॐ

MY PRAYER FOR YOU: Dear Lord, please don't let the enemy of this woman's soul make her feel as if the train has pulled out of the station and she missed it. Let her know You acknowledge her pain, I pray. Comfort her bruised soul. Show her how much You love her where she's at today, and that You have beautiful, wonderful—good—plans for her. Amen, my King!

11

The Amazing and The Tragic

MY GROWTH AND PROGRESS through infertility would have been greatly hindered had I not utilized what I fondly call my Support Structure. Conversely, I know people who have made use of what appeared to be sound support and help only to be caught up in self-destructive lies, which reminds me of one of the most tragic things I've ever witnessed.

I once found myself accompanying my husband on a business trip to a stunningly beautiful, European country. On one of our excursions, we were moving from one portion of a clean, efficient train station to another, and there she was: the girl I will never forget.

She appeared to be in her late teens or early twenties, with beautiful, flowing hair. Slim and lovely, she was scrunched on the side of the stairwell, leaning against the wall—oblivious to those walking around her—in the process of injecting what was most likely heroin into her left forearm's bruised, puffy vein. I froze, and Brad gently—but firmly—moved me forward. He knew my instincts would be to try and engage with her in the hope of providing life-changing care. He *also* knew the girl would viciously fight anyone who tried to intervene while she was in the middle of getting what she wanted more than anything else in the world at that moment.

Desperate for a fix, this woman-child was oblivious to the magnificent countryside and culture around her, or of anything good. It was all about the fix. She had to have it and nothing else mattered at that moment.

My mind was whirling as we continued on our way. What was her name? Was there anyone in her life who cared about her? How could a girl so attractive, with such breathtaking beauty all around her, end up in a public stairwell jamming a needle full of garbage into herself?

Tragic!

And equally tragic is the fact that you and I can end up in a similar plight if we permit *anything* which is even slightly off in the spiritual realm to lodge itself into our support structure as we seek to navigate the trials of life. Let me explain.

We previously addressed the existence of three enemies that work against us: Satan, the world, and our flesh. Did you know any one of those three can infiltrate what *may appear* to be an appropriate tool for help, only to end up turning on us in the same way as a fiercely addicting, illicit drug? And unlike the girl in the stairwell who *knew* she had a problem, we may not even know—between our fixes—that we're allowing a substance into our minds and hearts just as deadly as heroin.

What does this mean? Simply this: our support structures can be amazing—or tragic. Let's see what we can do to make them what God, the lover of our souls, intended.

THE AMAZING—GOD HIMSELF

For the Christ follower, the main means of support is his or her relationship, fellowship, and communication with God. Because God knows what is best for us (see Jeremiah 29:11) and loves us so much (see Romans 5:8), He provided us with the Holy Spirit—who actually indwells each believer (see John 14:17)—and gave us His Word to be our guide (see Psalm 119:105). God provided us with the most powerful means of support in the whole of creation: Himself.

This is insanely fabulous!

Perhaps what you're reading here is new to you, and you're afraid to be intimate with God. If so, I understand. God is so holy, all-knowing, and frightening, really. How can we be intimate with Him? By this: simply telling Him we want to be and asking Him to teach us and show us how. Oh, friend! He will! (see James 4:8)

If we are not relying primarily on God and His Word to help us through our infertility battles, we're tragically emulating the girl at the train station. You may be able to coast along for a while with the support of your husband, friends, pastor, counselor, or a doctor, perhaps; but the day will come when you'll hit rock bottom and they will not be around, or *able*, to supply you adequately. *Nothing else is even close to being an adequate substitute for God, or your time alone with Him and His Word.*

As we consider God (our Father), Christ (the perfect Savior who suffered more than any of us), and the Holy Spirit (the Comforter sent to indwell every believer), we'll recognize we *possess* more support than we could ever *use* right there.

The Apostle Paul wrote: "Blessed be the God and Father of our Lord Jesus Christ, who has blessed us with every spiritual blessing in the heavenly places in Christ" (Ephesians 1:3).

This is a verse we should never be able to read without being somewhat stunned. As an adopted child of God, you have been given *every spiritual blessing* in the heavenly places in Christ. Simply put: God has already given us what we so often beg Him for and fail to use.

※

When in high school, my childhood dream suddenly and unexpectedly came true. I became the owner of a delightful horse named Java. What a *love* I had for that animal! I spent time with my trail-loving horse nearly every day. But I was perplexed to observe how the owners of beautiful horses boarded at the nearby farm rarely took them out and enjoyed them.

As Ephesians 1:3 challenged my thinking, I began to think about the spiritual blessings God had given to me in terms of horses. Spiritually, I had an empty corral and God filled it with "horses" when I entrusted my life to His Son. There were several: the pretty one with the white blaze was named Love. The one near the watering trough was Peace. Then, there was the roan named Joy and the clean-limbed bay, Strength. The longer I looked, the more there were to see.

I own them; God graciously *gave* them to me. So even though these spiritual blessings are in my possession, am I faithfully saddling up Peace and taking him for a ride? Do I put these horses to *work* and enjoy having them? Or am I like the owners of the horses where Java was boarded who had valuable possessions but never or rarely used them?

Are the spiritual horses God has given to us getting regular exercise? Or do they stand in the corral day after day, waiting with pricked ears for us to come and get them but instead see us walking around the corral fence asking God for some spiritual horses to ride? What a picture!

We possess perfect, flawless support from God. Praise His holy name! Every Christian—not just a few—are in receipt of *every* spiritual blessing. God has given us Himself and the Bible. It takes action on our part, however, to use that support. How? By studying God's Word, praying, hanging out and delighting in Him, and obeying Him. That, my friend, is *amazing*.

YOUR HUSBAND

Next in our support structures should be our husbands. As a man of God and my spouse, Brad offers the sympathy, concern, and broad shoulder to cry on I often need. My hope, of course, is that your husband is the same type of shelter and refuge for you. But what if he isn't? And what would I need to do if Brad ceased being the type of support I needed him to be? What if you're the stronger of the two? Should we then sidestep our husbands and select another person for the next layer of our support structure?

No matter what our husbands are like, or how strong we ourselves may be, we must make them the vital, next segment of our support structures. Our relationships with our husbands—for better or for worse—are so important that I devote an entire chapter to the subject. In the meantime, while you are either in the process of developing your support structure or perhaps beginning to think you should be remodeling it, please reflect and pray about ways in which you can be improving your *friendship* with your husband. Proactively seek ways in which you can permit him to encourage and help you, even as you seek to be of encouragement and support to him.

CHRISTIAN WOMEN

After my husband, I then have a couple of special Christian women who complete my well-functioning support structure. In their shadows, so to speak, are some amazing men of God—their husbands. Before I go any further, however, I must humbly address a danger area.

Once we start utilizing any human beings other than our spouse as a part of our support structure, there are inherent risks. And Satan knows how to capitalize on our weaknesses. I will address several, but this one comes first: Do not have any man other than your husband or father (if he is a Christ follower) as a part of your support structure. The *only* exception to this is when a godly man is a part of *your husband's* support structure, and even then do not share, pray, or talk with him one on one. Many well-intentioned ministry efforts have ended in emotional or sexual impurity no one would have believed possible. If you fail to put an adequate boundary around yourself, it's similar to taking repeated, little shots of heroin to the vein. You may feel some temporary relief or comfort in the process, but it *will* hurt yourself and others in the long run.

The same thing is true regarding any non-Christian woman, friend, or relative you have in your support structure. No matter how comfortable you are with her or how much you cherish her insights, people we love or respect who do not have a personal, vibrant relationship with Jesus Christ are incapable of giving us the absolute best in support.

Candidates for our one-on-one support structure need to be women so deeply in love with Jesus Christ that their lives—though perhaps marred by pain—are a beautiful, compelling sign which continually points us to spiritual excellence and creates in us a thirst and appetite for God and His Word.

I've shared a great deal with you about trusting God, practicing obedience, and focusing on a worthy life goal; however, this has not insulated me from failing to remember every important spiritual lesson or truth, or caused me to automatically practice what I've learned every minute of every day. At times I experience fear or become discouraged with God's timetable. Although these times are never peaceful, it has been tremendously helpful for me to have godly friends who care enough to pick up on my spiritual discord and come alongside me with loving encouragement. They're humble and equipped not just to make me feel better but also probe my mind and heart and always, *always* wash me in the life-giving water of God's Word.

BUT I DON'T HAVE FRIENDS LIKE THAT!

I recognize you may not have the kind of friend or friends you need. If you don't have any Christian women you are close to, something is wrong unless, perhaps, you've been a believer for only a short time. Whether you live out in the sticks or are new in a community, you should be involved in a local, Bible-believing church. Trying to find Christian friends without being physically involved in a church family is like a fisherman trying to catch fish out of his bathtub.

If you're lacking a godly woman in your life, please ask God to give you one. Then be willing to be vulnerable and go out in search of her.

SIGNS OF FALSEHOOD MIXING WITH TRUTH

What are some signs of the tragic nipping at our heels? How can we separate the good from the bad?

If you'll recall our earlier example of the apprentice who wanted to learn how to differentiate real jade from counterfeit, remember the master taught him to become so familiar with authentic jade that the moment a counterfeit piece was placed in his hands he would *know* it was fake. We must be intimately familiar with the truth of God's Word so as to immediately recognize falsehoods. Lies can be so cleverly woven into truth that even a seasoned lover of the Bible can become misled. Even if we aren't enjoying perfect recall of scripture, we can (and should) search the Bible to see what God has to say about a matter.

One of the surest methods for recognizing a cleverly designed falsehood is this: If what you are reading, hearing, or pondering is giving you a pass on following any of God's commands or instructions for believers—whether it's viewed as a permanent pass or a temporary one—then it is tragically false. Together, we could probably come up with many examples, but here are three:

✹ "You can't fully forgive someone until that person has come to a full understanding of the depth of the hurt or damage he or she caused you." *Temporary pass: somebody has to come around or realize something before you can be obedient (but see Ephesians 4:32).*

✹ "Only after you've learned to love yourself can you truly follow God's command to love Him and to love others." *Temporary pass: you have work to do before you can be obedient (but see Matthew 22:37).*

✹ "You have to do what's right for you." *Permanent pass: God and His written commands, teachings, and/or principles aren't a match for the need of the moment. It's impractical to be obedient (but see Judges 21:25).*

Equally important for instantly recognizing cleverly designed falsehoods is this: If what you are reading, hearing, or pondering *deviates even slightly* from what God has communicated and preserved in the Bible about Himself, His Word, the human condition, His children, consequences of actions or inactions, or anything else, it is dangerously and tragically false. Consider some excuses you might hear (or tell yourself):

✻ "The Bible is outdated and old-fashioned. It isn't relevant to our lives today." *God says: "All Scripture is inspired by God and profitable for teaching, for reproof, for correction, for training in righteousness" (2 Timothy 3:16).*

✻ "If God is good, why does He let such horrible things happen?" *God says: "God is Light, and in Him there is no darkness at all" (I John 1:5).*

✻ "I know the book of Romans talks about all things working together for good for somebody, but it certainly can't be talking about *my* good." *God says: "God causes all things to work together for good to those who love God, to those who are called according to His purpose" (Romans 8:28).*

STRUCTURAL ENGINEERING

Believe it or not, this ties into our subject (if you're familiar with rebar, pardon the pun). How would you feel about crossing a bridge if you found out the individual who designed it wasn't a very good engineer? Or actually wasn't an engineer at all but someone who *posed* as an engineer? You might think twice before traversing the structure.

Jesus shared something alarming about *foundations* with a large crowd of people one day—something every structural engineer would understand. Remember first who Jesus is, though: *God the Creator in human flesh (see Colossians 1:15-16).*

The One who intimately knew and created physics used a physical illustration to make a critically important spiritual point easy for us to understand. No matter how brilliantly something is designed or constructed, it's not going to stand up to the test of time if it isn't built on a solid foundation:

> Therefore, everyone who hears these words of Mine and acts on them, may be compared to a wise man who built his house on the rock. And the rain fell, and the floods came, and the winds blew and slammed against that house; and yet it did not fall, for it had been founded on the rock. Everyone who hears these words of Mine and does not act on them, will be like a foolish man who built his house on the sand. The rain fell, and the floods came, and the winds blew and slammed against that house; and it fell—and great was its fall. (Matthew 7:24-27)

Support structures—our foundations in life—can be either amazing or tragic. God gives us the choice.

༚

Based on what we've covered, are there any areas within your support structure—your foundation—which may contain weaknesses? Are you willing to identify and eradicate, with the help of God's Holy Spirit, any areas of compromise? What tools are you using to determine whether something you are hearing, reading, or pondering may be a mixture of truth and falsehood?

❧

MY PRAYER FOR YOU: Father, if it is what will most honor You, I ask this cherished reader in wait for a child be given the gift of motherhood. May wisdom and discernment flow from You, enabling her to diligently build her life on the Solid Rock of Jesus Christ, not only for *her* benefit (which I so desire!) but so her child or children will grow up with a front-row seat observing, firsthand, a life solidly anchored in the amazing.

12

Spaghetti Sauce Days

HAVE YOU EVER had a morning when you felt so in tune with God and so full of joy in Him your heart felt as though it would burst? I was having such a morning one day, and it was indescribable. I was carrying out my household duties with singing and praise (somewhat unusual, for me), and felt as though I had, at last, "mounted up with wings as eagles" (see Isaiah 40:31). God had been so free with His blessings towards me and I was amazed at the number of answers to prayer I was seeing. It almost seemed as if God had come right down beside me and said, "Isn't it sweet to trust in Me?"

The Lord had patiently seen me through many hurdles, and I knew in my heart He was taking the "extra time" for us to have a family because He was careful, wise, and loved us so dearly. The Bible verse about God causing all things to work together for good (Romans 8:28) had become my encouragement and bedrock. It now flowed frequently and beautifully through my thinking. And because of it all, I was full of praise and trust that wonderful day!

This same morning it came to my attention one of our friends was sick. I felt inspired to fix dinner for the family and made arrangements. My large crockpot was soon simmering fragrantly with spaghetti sauce. As I added the spices, I found myself praying the love of Christ could somehow be tasted by the family members, as they didn't know Jesus as their Lord and Savior. I kept singing and practically gliding around the house, with thoughts attuned to my wonderful Lord.

A few hours later, I was on my way to deliver the sauce the short distance to our friends' home. With the crock of sauce setting on the floor of the car, I cautiously made my second corner. While doing so, the gas pedal suddenly seemed to press down of its own accord. And what do you think happened next? *Yes!* The goofy car, empowered by a good shot of fuel, seemed to take on a life of its own. To my horror, the crock of spaghetti sauce began to tip over. With one hand, I quickly reached over and grabbed the top of the container before it could fall, while hurriedly pulling over to the side of the road. Once stopped, I saw that some sauce had most *beautifully* slopped over the rim of the crockpot and spilled onto the carpeting.

I can't believe this! I inwardly fumed.

Sure, I could have found a safer way to transport the sauce. But that failed to explain the gas pedal problem. What had *happened*, anyway?

Words again fail to describe the feelings I was having, only this time they had *nothing* to do with rejoicing. Anger boiled up within me, and it was directed at *God*.

"Lord, why this?" I questioned. "You *knew* this was going to happen all the time I was praising You, and that's not fair! I was doing all this cooking and stuff for *You* to begin with! And it isn't as though I made this spaghetti sauce to take to a Satanic potluck, You know!"

Still upset, I drove back home and carried the crockpot into the house before beginning the laborious task of cleaning out the mess in the car. (Spaghetti sauce does wonders for carpeting, so that little chore went far in cheering me up.)

Next came cleaning off the lid and crockpot and surveying the remaining sauce. The amount left unscathed was likely enough for the family's meal, but what if it wasn't? I fretted over that possibility before deciding to play it safe and adding the portion of sauce reserved for our own dinner to the sauce awaiting delivery. *Great,* I mused in self-pity. *Now I have to figure out what to make us for supper tonight.*

With everything again organized, I began to feel ashamed for my instant anger. What was my problem, anyway? When would I ever learn to stop getting angry with God? Why had my joy and praise vanished so suddenly? My communion with the Lord had been so special, so genuine! How could I let such a small thing ruin my intimacy with God? And why couldn't I just take things like spaghetti sauce tipping over in stride, or with a little humor? I was not pleased with myself, but still inwardly trying to fathom why God seemingly put His finger right down on that car's accelerator.

My conscience was flaying me, and I knew I had to put my irritation aside and ask God's forgiveness for my rash anger. The more I recalled the beautiful intimacy He had shared with me that morning, the sicker at heart I became for my later thoughts toward Him. Thoroughly humbled, I confessed what I had done was horribly wrong and that I was grieved for having sinned. Since I had come to believe God is the giver of all our possessions, I acknowledged the spaghetti sauce was technically His to begin with, and if *He* wanted to let the car *He* gave us have a gas attack and spill some of *His* sauce, then I would try to accept that.

I seriously thought things over and concluded if Romans 8:28 was *really* true, then it would cover not only big things like infertility, but minor disasters such as spilled spaghetti sauce. This concept made me somewhat nervous, and very much humbled. I found myself praying again and experiencing peace. It wasn't long before I picked up the crockpot and headed toward the door. *If at first you don't succeed, try and try again...*

Just then, our only phone at the time—a land line—rang.

Never had the ringing of a telephone seemed to carry such incredible significance as at that moment. The sound of it stopped me in my tracks. Goosebumps ran over me when the second ring came, followed by a crystal clear understanding, which I instantly knew was from God: *You wouldn't have been home to answer the phone if the spaghetti sauce hadn't tipped over.*

A fast, silent prayer shot heavenward. "Father! Is this an important call You wanted to make sure I didn't miss, so You allowed the spaghetti sauce to spill?" I actually trembled as I set my things down and thought with amazement of how Romans 8:28 could apply to *spaghetti sauce*. I thanked the Lord with awe and rushed to pick up the phone.

A familiar voice said, "Hi, June!"

My sudden, wonderful expectations about doing something great for the Lord (such as encouraging a friend in need) popped like a balloon. It was none other than my friend Tamara. Without meaning to, she had become a source of pain for me. She would call me on a regular basis and ask, "Has your period started yet?" You can imagine how overjoyed I was to receive such calls. She was concerned about our infertility problem; enough (so it seemed to me) to bring it up *every* time we visited. I had grown quite weary of this pattern, but God seemed determined to keep this nonbeliever in my life, and this appeared to be her role.

Tamara was expecting a baby, and I felt I owed it to her to ask how she had been feeling. I then heard about her latest doctor's appointment before she suddenly said:

"I'm sure sorry you can't seem to get pregnant."

Almost immediately, I could feel my blood pressure climbing. I began thinking, *Thanks, God! You let the spaghetti sauce tip over so I could stand here and listen to this?!*

"That's okay, Tamara. If God wants us to get pregnant, we'll get pregnant." I said this as cheerfully as possible, but even I didn't miss the "let's talk about the weather next" tone in my voice.

"I suppose so. But it's been such a long time for you."

I acknowledged that painful truth before sharing my belief that God's timing and God's ways were best, and what Brad and I really wanted. Tamara was generally uncomfortable any time God or Christ entered into our conversations, and I was hoping my truthful remark would work two ways. That it would cause her to stop pestering me about our lack of family and make her uncomfortable with the subject, since God seemed to be playing a major role in it.

"I hope so," Tamara said with dreadful persistence. "I'd hate to think you were... *obsessed* about getting pregnant. Do you know what I mean?"

Am I hearing right? I asked myself. This was pretty insensitive stuff, even from someone who was a bold communicator.

"Well," I said hesitantly, "I don't think I am. I'm trusting God—"

Before I could even finish speaking, Tamara, in a sweet voice said, "I'd hate for it to be *so important* to you that you couldn't *handle* it if you couldn't get pregnant."

I stood breathless, paralyzed by what I'd just heard. *Why didn't she just shut up?*

"I mean," she continued, "it's very possible you might never be able to have your own baby."

I wanted to scream and fought back angry tears. Shaking with emotion, I silently prayed for God's help. How cruel! How unbelievably cruel! I couldn't understand why I was having to endure this horrible experience. Still feeling numb after the phone call, I dried my tears, delivered the spaghetti sauce, and came home.

Over and over her words echoed in my mind.

It's very possible you might never be able to have your own baby.

I sat down on the couch.

I'd hate to think you were obsessed about getting pregnant.

Those awful statements, delivered in a tone I interpreted to be smugness, almost gloating; sugar-coated by "concern" as only a woman can do.

What I have to share next isn't easy. In fact, I tried to come up with ways to leave this chapter out of the book or soften the account of what next took place. But I know God, in His sovereignty, intended for you to know the ugly truth.

Seemingly out of nowhere, a sudden, intense hatred for Tamara consumed me.

Within an hour, I had gone all the way from being excited about doing something for God to actually relishing the thought of someone I knew going to hell. At that moment in time, with every ounce of my being, I hated Tamara's pregnancy. I hated her calls. I hated *her*. Her eternal state didn't concern me in the least. God's desires were not mine, and I told myself I simply didn't care.

These heartless thoughts were mine for several moments. But soon, tears trickled down my cheeks as I loathed myself for *again* failing to come through a tough situation in a way which was honoring to Christ. What a rotten friend I was! And such a horrible, pitiful representation of true Christianity. Why, oh *why* should I keep trying to be pure when all I ever did was fall flat on my face?

I slid to my knees. "Lord," I cried out. "I'm so sorry! Please forgive me! But I can't help the way I feel. How could Tamara be so mean to me? What did I ever do to deserve this?" My prayer seemed to echo hollowly off the walls. I knew I should be scared to death for Tamara's well-being. She didn't know Christ; she was spiritually lost.

But, really, I found myself again reasoning selfishly, *how could I? How could anyone care for someone who was so insensitive?* Remorse began slipping away and resentment gained a fresh foothold. *How could Tamara call me her friend,* I wondered, *and deliberately rub my nose in the fact she's pregnant, I want to be, and very possibly never will be?* With friends like that who needed *enemies?* For that matter who needed Tamara?

Certainly not me! I decided I'd had *enough*; I was finished with my prayers for her. *So what if she went to hell,* I thought? That was her problem not mine. I resolved to spend my time and energies on more appreciative people.

❧

Twisted and awful as they were, those were my intentions. When Brad got home from work, I told him the whole account. There was no raving or crying; I was very calm and controlled. Perhaps Brad was beginning to wish (for the first time in his life) that I *would* cry. This dreadfully soft, matter-of-fact declaration of abandonment was far more alarming than tears or ungoverned outbursts. And from the depths of my heart, I meant it. Tamara was out of my life. *Forever.*

In my mind, I also coldly challenged God: *Romans 8:28 certainly back-fired here, didn't it?*

※

Seeing Brad battle this latest development was interesting. I was relieved that he was becoming angry with Tamara also. You see, in my state of sinning, I didn't *want* Brad to encourage me. I didn't *want* him to say I misunderstood her motives. I didn't *want* him to share any biblical truths about unconditional love or to defend Tamara's actions if she was being insensitive because she didn't know the Lord. I wanted to be mad, and my fervent desire was for Brad to understand the depth of my hurt and be angry too!

Well, he was mad all right. He fumed pretty well himself. How could anyone be so cruel to his wife? he asked. What was Tamara's problem, anyway?

I felt *much* better about my own sin when Brad was struggling so mightily with his! Brad's anger, however, was short lived. It was like a brightly lit torch that suddenly fizzled and died.

"June, this isn't right." Sadness and conviction in his voice underscored each word.

Of course I knew it wasn't right, but it sure felt good to me.

"Oh, come on Brad. *Let* me be angry. I have a right to! Tamara put the knife in my heart and twisted it. Nobody's ever hurt me that badly," I said, choking back a sob.

We sat together in silence. All throughout my childhood I had been trained to love and care for others. I could feel the Holy Spirit tugging at my heart and fought it. "Do not grieve the Holy Spirit of God, by whom you were sealed for the day of redemption" (Ephesians 4:30) flashed through my mind. *Stop the verses, God! I don't want to hear any!* Several minutes ticked by. I could sense Brad's spirit continuing to soften.

"June, this is really hard for me too. I don't enjoy people hurting you. And I don't understand why God allowed you to get a phone call like that. But for some reason He did."

I recall sitting on the couch, deeply resenting what I was hearing. Brad's brow was furrowed in thought, and for a while it seemed as though he had forgotten I was there. This did *not* thrill me for it generally meant Brad was about to become excruciatingly practical—the *last* thing I wanted just then! What I longed for was to ride high on the waves of bitterness and revenge. All my life I had tried to be good. I wanted to be free of that for a while.

My fears, however, were soon realized. Brad, ever the practical thinker, threw me a funny look and asked if I had been praying for Tamara lately. I love my husband, but frequently hate his questions, "Yes, I have," I said. He looked slightly puzzled.

"*How* have you been praying for her?"

"What do you mean?" I asked without bothering to mask my annoyance.

"In what way have you been praying for Tamara?"

After thinking it over for a moment, I slowly admitted, "Well, I've been praying there would be a change in our relationship. You know, that it would become more personal, more intimate. And through it she would come to a saving knowledge of Jesus Christ."

"So you've been praying for a more intimate relationship with Tamara?"

"Yes," I answered before adding, "I should have been more specific in my prayers because what I've ended up with is a more intimately *painful* relationship with her." Not only did Brad choose to ignore my rancid sarcasm, he went so far as to suggest we talk a little longer about Tamara.

"How many close friends—girlfriends—does Tamara have, June?"

His question made me wary. I had a fleeting premonition as to where this conversation could lead, and I didn't like it.

"Well, Tamara doesn't really have what I would call girlfriends," I said slowly. "She has several acquaintances, but as far as close friends go, I'm not sure."

"Who would you say is Tamara's closest friend?" Brad probed in seeming innocence.

"From whose perspective?" I returned in irritation. "Hers or mine?"

"Hers."

I sighed heavily and looked at the man. He was being most sincere.

"I suppose that I'm about Tamara's closest friend." The words sounded profane, and I could feel a wave of crimson working its way across my face. "And I've been too frustrated to even speak much with her lately. Oh, that's terrible!"

"And here's Tamara," Brad stated practically, "at one of the most exciting times of her life. Who does she have to share it with? I don't think she has a close, intimate relationship with her own mom. So who, really, does Tamara have to share her excitement with?"

"Jacob." I responded feebly.

"Oh, June! I mean girls... *women!* Men really don't get into all that baby talk like women do. Who can she talk girl talk with?"

"Well, Brad," I flared angrily, "it's Tamara's own rotten fault if she doesn't have a big group of girlfriends to be intimate with! If she would be *nice* to people, she would have friends like the rest of the world. She ought to be smart enough to figure *that* out!"

A strained silence settled over us.

"June," Brad ventured tenaciously, "didn't Tamara tell you at one point in time she's never had any close friends in her life? That she always felt like a misfit?"

"Yes."

"So, she's never really learned *how* to be close friends with anyone. She may not even know how to go about it. What do you think? Could that be a possibility?"

"I guess." I breathed out in some resentment.

"I could be way out in left field, but this idea just occurred to me. Is it possible Tamara's making a genuine effort to be more intimate with you but just kind of goofed it up? And the more she said, the worse it got? What do you and her have in common besides being married? Babies! She's going to have one, and you *want* to have one. It could be a simple attempt of her reaching out for a more intimate relationship with you and unwittingly hurting your feelings in the process." Excitement was beginning to grow in Brad, and I didn't know whether or not to become a part of it.

Was Brad so grossly optimistic that he could twist this awful situation into something like a friend reaching out for a more personal relationship? Or was I a huge fool, and God was insistently laying out Romans 8:28 for me again?

Questions, questions! I didn't want questions *or* options. I just wanted to have a rotten attitude in peace; but Brad's thoughts bothered me. Oh, my goodness! What if he were right?

Naaww, *it couldn't be!* Tamara the innocent victim and *me* the horrible friend?

Why did Brad have to come up with a crazy idea like that, anyway? Why didn't he and God just let up on me for a while, so I could indulge myself in anger toward Tamara for at *least* a few days or weeks? Was that really asking for too much?

But I found myself thinking about Tamara and her earlier admission of having had no close friends in her life. What if *I* was the one who was wrong? Could this whole mess have been an attempt by Tamara to be a genuinely more caring person? As an actual answer to *my own* prayers?

Ouch!

Could Tamara have been reaching out for a closer relationship, one where I could become a better friend, who would then have greater freedom to share Christ with her? *As if Christ still would want to have anything to do with me after this day!*

Despite my self-centered ugliness, I considered further. God *deeply* loved Tamara. I knew that! And Christ *died* for her. As a child of God, I recognized I was commanded to love—even my enemies (see Matthew 5:44). So whether Brad's train of thought was on or off track, it didn't matter in God's Book.

"If you love Me, you will keep My commandments" (John 14:15).

❧

Brad shared a few more thoughts with me and assured me of his love and sympathy. His understanding and desire to trust the Lord made my heart well up with gratitude for the man God had chosen for my mate. As I began to relax a little, the tears came freely. It was a relief and partial surrender. After my cry, I leaned against Brad, apologized, and thanked him for what he had done. Nevertheless, I still had some doubts.

"Brad, I'm still not sure about this," I admitted. "The thought of hanging in there with Tamara frightens me. I don't want to get hurt again. But regardless of whether God revealed to you how things are with her, or if you're shooting in the dark, I *know* God wants me to have a deep love for her."

Brad sat quietly and let me talk.

"But I guess I want to have assurances from God that Tamara wasn't just trying to be mean to me," I said. By the expression on my husband's face I knew what he was about to say, but I continued, "I *know* it shouldn't matter, or that it doesn't change my responsibility to Tamara; it's just I got hurt so very badly. I need some *extra* reassurance from God."

"Such as?" Brad asked.

"Like, well, I want to put out a sort of test before the Lord, I guess."

Brad doubted the merits of my idea. With a definite lack of enthusiasm, he inquired as to just what kind of test I had in mind.

"For Tamara maybe to call me by tomorrow night," I explained. "And for a miracle to happen where we just talk like two friends and *nothing* she says hurts my feelings. And babies or pregnancy aren't mentioned, just once! And that I have a *truly* enjoyable visit with her."

A hibernating bear could have sensed Brad's doubts. For all his encouragement, he still had his own struggles with Tamara's drilling questions and the subject of our infertility. I knew he was thinking: *How could the two of them talk without that subject coming up? And June's feelings are too raw; she's like a powder keg. Besides, is putting such a thing before the Lord even right?*

I prayed about it at length and did put that very test before God, begging for His mercy and understanding. The Lord didn't need to prove anything to me, but He honored my test just the same. Tamara called the very next morning.

❧

What an absolute joy she was to speak with! We had a truly wonderful visit! And all my terms were met.

❧

As a child, I was fascinated by the Bible stories I was taught with beautiful, flannel backgrounds and paper cut-out characters used by my mother in her Good News Clubs and during Vacation Bible School. Some of my favorite stories were from the Old Testament. I recalled the account of fire falling down from heaven to burn up Elijah's sacrifice (see I King 18), the terrifying plagues God brought upon Egypt (see Exodus 7-12), Moses and his experience with the burning bush (see Exodus 3), and the parting of the Red Sea by Jehovah God for the children of Israel as they fled Pharaoh and his armies (see Exodus 14). But what I had just experienced—my grotesque misjudgment of a friend and bitterness towards her; my inappropriate request of the Lord to honor my test about Tamara; and the miracle that followed—was incomprehensible to me.

The miracle God performed in that situation was every bit as powerful as the miracles of the Bible I knew and loved.

I was thrilled by—and afraid of—what had happened. The test proved beyond any doubt God had indeed revealed to Brad the true status of Tamara's heart. *She* was the one reaching out in love and concern. I was the one so wrapped up in myself that I had absolutely no discernment as to how the Lord had been at work in this young woman's heart. I had completely missed the fact that God had been answering my own prayers for Tamara to become more open to an intimate relationship.

The greater miracle than the honoring of my test, perhaps, was God not severely punishing me for my hardness of heart or lack of faith. I recalled the biblical account of the earth opening up and swallowing people whose transgressions were certainly no greater than mine (see Numbers 16; it will raise your hair!). I immediately received a much deeper appreciation and understanding of God's mercy. His power filled me with awe, and all my thoughts for Tamara were transformed into what they should have been all along: genuine love and concern.

The result? Well, what do you think? I was bouncing off the walls! God was personally merciful to me in the most amazing way! He performed a miracle for me that I didn't deserve in the least.

I wanted to rush out and tell the whole world, *"You will never believe what God taught me through a tipped over crockpot of spaghetti sauce, people!"* But God was far from being finished with the matter.

❦

Two days later, I was sitting at my friend Paige's dining room table. The two of us were having a menu and meal planning session for an upcoming camping trip with our husbands. Vicki, Paige's mom, was visiting that day, which enabled me to get a bit reacquainted with her. After a while, Vicki went to one of the back rooms to watch her favorite soap opera while Paige and I started our camping plans. We didn't stay on task for long because I just *had* to share with her what God had done with the spaghetti sauce. So off I went into my long-winded account of the day's beginning. While describing my second attempt to deliver the spaghetti sauce, Vicki came out to the dining room and began listening. As I was sharing the details of my experience on the phone with Tamara, Vicki's eyes snapped brightly.

"What an *awful* thing!" she exclaimed. As my tale continued, Vicki grew angry and indignant over what Tamara had said and commented, "Well, don't waste any time on *her* again!"

I encouraged Vicki to hear the end of the story. It was meaningful to not only be able to share with Paige the incredible miracle and spiritual victory God had given me but also that her mother—who didn't have a personal relationship with Jesus—was hearing a testimony of God's power to change hateful attitudes. After I concluded, Paige's mother said, "Well, June, that's good. I'm really glad you know God and want to do what's right. I do too. I know what a person has to do to go to heaven."

Vicki's last remark struck me as odd; it almost seemed to be an unrelated thought or topic and caught my full attention. So to my surprise, I found myself following up on it. "And what do you believe that is?" I asked.

She paused only a moment before replying, "Why, to go to heaven, you've got to be nice to other people. And do a lot of good things."

Paige, a fairly new believer in Christ, sat mutely watching the conversation unfold. My heart began pounding furiously.

That was certainly one of Satan's most popular deceptions. But how could I tell that to Vicki? I didn't want to hurt her feelings or say anything that might make her feel dumb.

Satan, I realized, was tempting me to keep quiet when God had provided a wide open door to share a critically important truth with Vicki. I briefly considered the temptation to keep quiet. With that very week's disaster all too fresh in my mind I was fearful of how consistently I messed things up. *Where's a pastor or more together Christian when you need one?* I wondered. But I silently prayed and asked God to help me share His Word.

"Vicki," I said gently. "In a way, I hate to tell you this, but that's wrong. Many people believe that, but it isn't the truth."

Her eyebrows arched quite beautifully, and she looked surprised. "It isn't?"

"No," I said softly, "look, here."

Before me were untouched sheets of paper for use in the meal planning and packing lists. For the first time in my life, I found myself sharing God's wonderful plan of salvation—of our sin and God's grace—in picture form.

First, I drew a picture of an old-fashioned scale and, using myself as an example, started drawing bricks on one side as I named off a smattering of sacrifices, good deeds, and community services I had performed.

"Wow!" Vicki said. "That really looks good!"

Then, on the other side of the scale, I began to add bricks for sins I had committed, such as lying, envy, and hatred. I said, "Many people think that if our good deeds outweigh our bad deeds, then we'll go to heaven when we die. But the Bible tells us in James 2:10 that *one* sin is all it takes to render us guilty before a perfect, holy God."

I briefly quoted Scripture verses the Lord brought to remembrance before drawing a picture of a great chasm, which separated sinful mankind from Holy God. I explained that only Christ, through His sacrifice on the cross, paid the price for our sins (I John 2:2). I explained how His burial and resurrection spanned that gulf and that Jesus is the way, the truth, and the life; no one can have access to God the Father, except through Him (John 14:6).

Vicki's eyes were huge.

"It's our belief in Jesus Christ and nothing else that saves us."

Vicki excused herself shortly thereafter. Paige and I looked at each other, slightly stunned. I finally managed a soft, "Praise God! What an unexpected opportunity!" Paige's eyes were as large as her mother's had been. She kept saying, "Wow, June! *Wow!*"

At last, we finished planning for the camping trip, and I began to leave. Vicki appeared once again, and we visited for a little while. Suddenly, she said, "June, I've never shared this with any of Paige's other friends before because I'm ashamed of it, I guess. But I feel I can tell you, and you won't think any less of me. I can't read."

At first, I was perplexed as to why Vicki chose to share something so personal and painful. We talked about it for a while longer before she wiped a tear from her eye.

"I want to thank you for telling me what you did about heaven and Christ today. And for the *way* you did it."

The full impact of her words took a few moments to hit me. Before I was out of the door I was trembling in deepest awe and thanksgiving. Because of what God had allowed me to go through with infertility and Tamara and the ultimate victory He gave me in that awful battle, I was able to present God's amazing plan of salvation to Paige's spiritually lost mom. *And God had moved me to share those truths verbally and in picture form to someone whom I hadn't even known was unable to read!*

❧

A few weeks later, Paige had the indescribable joy of leading her own mother into a personal relationship with Jesus Christ. Only short months after that, Vicki was diagnosed with cancer. She listened to the New Testament on audio. Her testimony and faith were not washed away in self-pity. She harbored no bitterness and shared Christ with those who would listen. She was given a few months to live and she lived each one of them for Christ.

❧

I traced the mystery of the part God allowed me to have in bringing Vicki to a saving knowledge of Jesus Christ, and it has humbled me greatly. I look back to a day when a tipped over crockpot of spaghetti sauce and my infertility pain caused me to bitterly question Romans 8:28.

It was a lesson I learned the hard way.

God's Word *will* stand forever (Isaiah 40:8), and those who question it will be silenced.

❧

God loved me enough to allow me to go through excruciating struggles so I could learn more about His sovereignty and the power and truth of His Word. He loved Vicki enough to let me experience difficulties He would use to draw her unto Himself! He loved Paige enough to allow a couple to suffer the pain of being childless so her mom could come to know the Lord before her death. And I knew He loved Tamara enough to one day lead her into a saving relationship with Him—which He did, several years later—despite her having such a problematic Christian friend.

It was at this point in my walk down the Path I found Romans 8:28 to be unquestionably true, along with the rest of God's Word:

And we know that God causes all things work together for good to them that love God, to them that are called according to His purpose.

ૐ

Some of the "good" mentioned in this verse will not be seen as readily as has been the case for my infertility, or the unexpected tipping over of a crockpot of spaghetti sauce one day. *But whether or not God allows us to see the good in each of our difficult situations this side of heaven does not mean the good is not happening.*

This, my friend, is breathtaking hope!

ૐ

As my trust has grown, my awareness of my failures before God has also grown. Perhaps my questions to God will be slower in coming. Perhaps my foolish ravings at God will cease as I grow to trust and know Him more, as I learn to be more obedient.

God led me to the Old Testament book of Job not long after this, where He admonished me gently yet with frightening power:

A messenger came to Job and said, "The oxen were plowing and the donkeys feeding beside them, and the Sabeans attacked and took them. They also slew the servants with the edge of the sword, and I alone have escaped to tell you." While he was still speaking, another also came and said, "The fire of God fell from heaven and burned up the sheep and the servants and consumed them, and I alone have escaped to tell you." While he was still speaking, another also came and said, "The Chaldeans formed three bands and made a raid on the camels and took them and slew the servants with the edge of the sword; and I alone have escaped to tell you." While he was still speaking, another also came and said, "Your sons and your daughters were eating and drinking wine in their oldest brother's house, and behold, a great wind came from across the wilderness and struck the four corners of the house, and it fell on the young people and they died; and I alone have escaped to tell you."

Then Job arose and tore his robe and shaved his head, and he fell to the ground and worshipped. And he said, "Naked I came from my mother's womb, and naked I shall return there. The LORD gave and the LORD has taken away. Blessed be the name of the LORD."

Through all this Job did not sin nor did he blame God. (Job 1:14-22)

It was as if God was saying to me, "My child, you have been a slow learner, but you have been learning. You've come to understand important truths which you needed to grasp in order to have a more joyful, victorious life in my Son. I have been pleased with your progress. However, it is time to deal with your foolish ravings towards Me. *I am God.*"

Yes, God *is* a heavenly Father to anyone who places his or her faith in Jesus Christ. But we must remember that *God is God.* Even on spaghetti sauce days.

MY PRAYER FOR YOU: Please allow this sweet woman to accept You and Your Word as truth. May You use my shame and failures to help her grasp and firmly hold onto what I was appallingly slow at doing: believing You are exactly who You say You are! I praise Your Holy Name.

13

Pursuing Pregnancy

HOW I WOULD LOVE to be a little bird perched on your shoulder right now! If you're like me, you may have perused this book's table of contents, skimming over chapter titles until you saw this one! *"Pursuing Pregnancy!" Yes! That's the chapter I care about the most. I'll read that one first and then go back and catch the others.* If you've done that, please know I've already laughed in understanding. I don't blame you in the least, but you've been caught!

On the other hand, if you're a straight arrow who has been steadfastly working your way through the chapters in order, I am so proud of you! Would you mind letting our friend who skipped straight to this chapter know she needs to go ahead and read this chapter, but then certainly detour back to the beginning? The truth, mercy, and power of God—and His downright shocking love for us (especially in light of our grievous shortcomings and failures)—is just too encouraging to miss.

So, "Pursuing Pregnancy" here we come!

❧

I want you to know I am all for this chapter; I cannot *tell* you how many people I have wished could read it, not the least of whom are doctors. The chapter's focus is to highlight what resources are available to the couple seeking to achieve what physicians call a "successful" pregnancy. *For this reason, it does not address all options we may have for becoming parents, such as adoption or foster parenting.*

Because God is in control of everything, as we know from the Bible, resolution of an infertility problem is not necessarily limited by one's financial resources. (Did I just hear an *Amen!?*)

If we look at infertility merely as a physical problem which must be addressed strictly in a physical manner—in other words, vainly leaving God out of our circumstance—those with greater financial capacity would be the fortunate elite and the remainder would be the disadvantaged, with very little hope of achieving a healthy pregnancy. God, however, has made it clear in His Word that He is what I call the Absolute Resource to the infertile woman or couple. *There is equal footing for resolution of infertility for all of God's children before His throne of grace and power.* Wow! That is so encouraging!

Perhaps in recognition of this, some Christians have rationalized that they shouldn't explore medical options for resolving their physical problem in their pursuit of parenthood. But is it wrong or a sign of weak faith in God to seek to educate ourselves and/or obtain help from doctors in an effort to resolve infertility?

When I found myself contemplating this question, God directed me—most interestingly—to the book of Joshua in the Old Testament. It served as a powerful reminder that

God, who is capable of doing any good thing, sometimes requires His beloved children to do things in a manner which is more difficult than may seem necessary. I encourage you to take your Bible and read Joshua 1–3. You'll notice when God directed Joshua to lead the children of Israel across the Jordan River—which was in full flood at the time—He required the priests leading the great company to actually *step into* the river. God had never asked anyone in recorded history prior to that moment to get their feet wet before He performed a miracle. Why did He require *that?*

We see another example of God's surprising way of doing things further back in Israel's history. In Exodus 13:17 we see how God miraculously led His people on a longer route than a map reveals was necessary after He released them from slavery in Egypt: "Now when Pharaoh had let the people go, God did not lead them by the way of the land of the Philistines, even though it was near." There was a direct route along the Mediterranean Coast to the Holy Land which would have been a journey of only a few *weeks*. The armies guarding and patrolling the route would have presented no problem to God, yet He led the children of Israel on a longer, less direct route. In time, it became apparent why God led them the way He did. They had a divine appointment to keep that changed the course of history and our lives today.

Yes, God is able to cause us to conceive and safely deliver a baby at any time. Despite this truth, it may be His desire for us to seek out medical help to see that blessing come to fruition. For us to assume God would not require any work on our part may be no different than if the children of Israel had decided to wait on the edge of the Jordan River to avoid getting their feet wet. And while to us it would seem more logical for us to get pregnant or carry a baby full term without having to explore possible resolutions for infertility, God may be leading us on a longer, more demanding route for reasons of His own.

SEEING A DOCTOR

If you have the ability to see a doctor in an effort to resolve an infertility problem, please be grateful, recognizing you are in a *very small group worldwide*. Even at that, most insurance plans don't cover infertility. Nonetheless, seeing a physician to resolve infertility is a resource some couples do have. If you and your husband are in this category, you may want to prayerfully consider making use of good medical technology if you're not doing so already. You'll see a significant portion of this chapter is devoted to this option and the critical doctor-patient relationship.

As Christians, we need not ignore technology. God Himself has allowed people to "increase in knowledge" (Daniel 12:4) Technology is not evil; it's what mankind does with it that can be good or evil. A worthwhile question to ask ourselves is whether we are using modern medicine with prayer and a true desire for God's will to be done? Or are we using it in an effort to thwart God's will for us: "We're going to get pregnant if it's the last thing we do!" Are we completely *against* using medical resources for treatment of a physical problem? As with all things, we need to strike a proper balance, and remember to allow God to saturate every area of our lives, including our pursuit of parenthood.

I know of couples with infertility who refuse to see a specialist about it. They state they *want* to have a baby but don't want to go "overboard" or "become obsessed by it." This line of reasoning made sense to me before discovering our own infertility. When reading about the enormous costs and frustrations some couples were incurring from their pursuit of conception, I was appalled. I wondered why they kept wasting their money and time. *If they want a baby so badly,* I wondered, *why don't they just adopt one?*

In my ignorance, I didn't realize there was no such thing as "just" adopting a baby. I was unaware of the true nature of the adoption process and hadn't stopped to think it was far more complicated and taxing—emotionally and financially—than it is. And I didn't understand why it was so important for couples to want to see what *their* offspring would be like, or for a woman or couple to have such an intense desire to experience pregnancy and childbirth together.

A review of our expenditures would reveal I now have a better understanding of those "crazy" couples spending so much time and money in an effort to have a successful pregnancy. Our own pursuit of parenthood, once I finally got going, has been very aggressive. We turned into one of those couples who have spent a good deal of time and money in an effort to have their "own kids." Although diligent pursuit of solving an infertility problem can be expensive, painful, and very frustrating at times, I've been grateful we've had the means and opportunity to try resolving that problem (even though we made significant sacrifices in order to survive, financially). We've been praying and asking God for children but also been out trying the doors of opportunity. My thought is, just as it makes no sense to ask God for spiritual growth but refuse to study our Bibles or practice obedience, we shouldn't ask God for children and never explore the medical options.

The day may well come, however, when Brad and I decide we need to stop. A particular procedure or method may prove to be more than we personally care to tackle. This doesn't alarm me for the simple reason that we are continually praying for God's guidance in our pursuit of parenthood. And should that day arrive, we'll be able to look at each other and agree, "We prayed about it and tried to do something through the means available. We gave it our best effort."

While those who are seeking medical assistance for infertility each have different situations, one thing we *should* share in common is exercising care as to who we're seeing and how we interact with them. If you are seeing a general practitioner or gynecologist for your infertility problem, it is highly probable you are not getting the *full* benefit of medical technology in the area of infertility. Infertility is a science of its own. There are specific treatments for the problem and specific physicians trained in this area. Making use of such specialists makes sense.

I wasted nearly a year with a doctor under a group health plan. When it came to treating infections, flu, and whatnot, he did just fine. But when I sincerely tried to discuss with him a possible infertility problem, he was of no help. I shared how long we had been trying to conceive and that I was occasionally having pregnancy-type symptoms, such as nausea, tender breasts and menstrual cycles which began later than usual. He responded by saying, "It sounds to me like you want to get pregnant too badly and might have a nerve problem." Let me say this: the gentleman may have been correct for all I know, but what was disturbing was his *quick judgment without checking anything out.*

This isn't to say doctors in group health plans are bad or that only infertility specialists can help you. But ask yourself:

"Is this the best place for someone experiencing problems with her (and/or her husband's) reproductive system to receive treatment?" If you're uncertain about how you should answer, it may be an indicator the answer could be *No*.

We decided to give the in-network physicians another try, and that's when things got even worse! This time, one of the doctors told me I was *lucky*. He said it was a real pain having to use birth control and that it must be *wonderful* not to have sex marred with the fear of producing babies. How insensitive! On the way to the car I thought, *Am I brainless? I just paid to have a doctor tell me how lucky I am to be infertile!*

Slowly, I was learning some valuable lessons:

Lesson #1: Seeking medical help for a physical problem is not a sign of weak faith in God.

Lesson #2: Just because you're a Christian or a nice person doesn't mean you have to trust or stick with your present physician.

Brad and I finally decided to seek medical help outside of our covered insurance in the hope of finding physicians who could better assist us, even though it would be a strain on our already tight budget. We began praying specifically for God to direct our steps. Before long, I was in the care of an exceptional gynecologist. We talked, he examined me and reviewed Brad's lab work; then we talked some more. I had questions; he answered them with sincerity and factually. He handled the obvious possible causes for infertility with me over a few brief months before recommending I see an infertility specialist he believed to be the best in the field. It was still disappointing to not yet be pregnant, but *very* encouraging to have someone finally really listen to me and care for me medically. One major frustration in my life had been eliminated.

God was faithful in answering our prayers about our physician. When the consultation with the infertility specialist took place, I knew right away he was tremendously knowledgeable. He queried us for every bit of information we could give, had Brad's lab results already on file and memorized, and reviewed the ovulation schedule the gynecologist had started me on. He took out a sheet of paper and wrote down the "plan of attack" he wanted to take. He explained the reasons why he wanted to check the things he would check, why he wanted to check them in the order he would check them, what was involved with each step, and what all the unfamiliar words and phrases meant. It seemed to be a very logical, practical plan after he explained it. Were we impressed? Yes. This was such a blessing compared to "Sounds like you want to get pregnant too bad and might have a nerve problem."

Before leaving that appointment (with helpful information sheets in hand), the doctor smiled and said, "Hopefully, we'll see you pregnant before long!" This basically summed up his goal. Here was a doctor whose goal matched ours—wanting to see *me* become a mother.

Of course, this is just one specialist out of many. I doubt all have the same drive and relentless pursuit of helping childless couples as our own infertility specialist, but I *do* believe most infertility specialists will be more alert, knowledgeable, helpful, and understanding than a general practitioner or gynecologist. The reason? It's their life's work. Even my excellent gynecologist knew an infertility specialist would have the edge on him in that area.

There's a disproportionate number of infertile couples and specialists to help them. Unless you live in or near an area with a large population, there is a good chance none exists within a one-hundred-mile radius of where you live. If there *is* one within commuting distance—even should the commute be inconvenient—I encourage you to prayerfully pursue seeing a specialist should you have the means to do so. I know of too many women who don't go to a specialist with their infertility problem and end up wasting time, money, and emotions on remedies that won't work. I was encouraged by the fact our doctor wanted to check such things as my husband's sperm count and mobility. He also checked my fallopian tubes (for blockages), my uterus, and my ovaries instead of mentally shrugging his shoulders and writing out a prescription for fertility pills. Such a prescription would have accomplished nothing except false hope if there were other problems.

There is a proper and logical order in which to examine the possible causes for a couple's infertility. Following a practical method of elimination can often save a couple *years* of effort and thousands of dollars in their pursuit of parenthood.

Many women are on fertility pills and aren't sure why. Some are having unnecessary operations when it turns out they had an easily correctible mucus problem (which costs only dollars to correct). There are too many people like Alisa who continue to see a doctor who for two years merely performed a pelvic examination each time she went in, telling her to be patient and just keep track of her time of ovulation. Through the prompting of a mutual friend, Alisa finally raised the courage to insist her doctor order lab tests on her husband's sperm. At first, her doctor *refused* her request. That, my friend, is unreasonable.

We cannot justify doggedly sticking with physicians who are not concerned with the patient's best interests. We cannot afford to be so polite or afraid to ask our doctors a few questions that we fail to receive the help needed for what *may* be a resolvable problem.

⁂

If you're receiving treatment for your infertility, does your treatment seem logical? Is your doctor laying out for you a reasonable, yet aggressive, schedule for determining what your complications are? Does your doctor focus his or her attention on both you and your husband, and how your body reacts with his sperm when united as a couple?

Whether you have a three- or four-hour commute to an infertility specialist or a relative short one, you *will* experience some frustrating days. You may expend major effort to get to an appointment to have your mucus or the lining of your uterus checked on a certain day of your cycle only to learn the timing was a little bit off, which means you'll have to retry the next month. You may go in with your husband to be artificially inseminated and find out your body hasn't produced *any* mucus and the procedure cannot be done. (I know I can't be the first person who stood in a parking lot and cried in frustration when this happened.) Nonetheless, even with gross inconveniences and several disappointments, Brad and I have not regretted seeing an infertility specialist. I do respectfully offer some tips I have learned over time, however, which may help as you interact with your physician:

Learn to talk to your doctor. Some patients are very good about asking key questions of their doctors and leave each appointment with all necessary issues addressed. Many of us, however, fail to do this. Despite good intentions and planned discussions, I have left a few appointments confused, or else I've believed I understood everything until that same evening

148

when Brad asked me about the appointment. Then I found myself answering his questions with phrases such as:

"I think he said…"
"I don't remember exactly what he told me about…"
"I forgot to ask about that…"
"I didn't ask because I hated to tie up his time…"

Does this sound a little familiar to you? If so, then you also have some bad habits to overcome.

Learn the art of asking questions. If you have questions left over from your last visit, or new questions for an upcoming one, *write them down.* Pull out your list of questions at the appointment and *refer* to it when you see the doctor. Don't worry what he or she might think. Your doctor will most likely be happy you aren't leaving with unanswered questions.

Doctors are supposed to be providing us with consultation. If your physician doesn't ask whether or not you have any questions, *you* need to open up the subject. Should your doctor speak too swiftly or in such complicated medical terms you have difficulty absorbing what he or she is telling you, stop the discourse and let him or her know. Remember, doctors *are* people. They may momentarily forget *you* are not an infertility specialist and don't know all the lingo. Training yourself to ask questions will benefit you only if you can understand and remember the answers. Make sure you understand *exactly* what your doctor is saying. Then, if you feel the need, write your answers down on the very sheet of paper or device on which you recorded your questions.

Be sure to ask about any tests, drugs, or procedures your doctor plans to utilize. When he or she is recommending a drug, ask about possible side effects. Fertility drugs affect some women very strongly, and it's beneficial to know in advance there might be hot flashes, dizziness, or emotionally charged hours during your treatment. If you have an upcoming test, don't be ashamed to ask if there is any accompanying discomfort with the test. It is the practice of some physicians to offer their patients a painkiller before some tests in order to help eliminate cramping.

If something your doctor has said or done is bothering you, let him or her know in a respectful, straightforward manner. While it isn't easy for most of us to do this, we owe it to ourselves and to our physicians. Your doctor, for example, may never have been told he or she gives the impression some procedures are simpler than they actually are. A good doctor will want to know how you're feeling and make any changes necessary to aid in improving his or her practice.

Should your doctor be unwilling to communicate with you in a kind, respectful manner, do not feel badly about seeking a replacement.

Evaluate your doctor's personality and schedule. Ideally, the patient-doctor relationship involves a certain degree of comfort, respect, and understanding by both parties. In the area of infertility, however, it's especially easy for a woman or couple to go beyond this stage to where they become psychologically dependent upon their physician. They may start off trusting their doctor. From there they may begin to want special attention or harbor unrealistic expectations of what their doctor should be doing or even what they think he or she should be like. If your doctor's mannerisms bother you, take time to evaluate his or her personality type. It may help you to understand him or her better, which will be beneficial as you interface with each other. Bear in mind your specialist may work many weekends, evenings, or holidays doing everything from seminars and surgery to offering free lectures.

Many couples blessed by medical options make the monumental decision to see a specialist to find out why they aren't conceiving and have high expectations for a quick cure. It's often an absolute shock when they find out how grueling the "finding and curing" process can be. Frustration and disillusionment can swiftly follow. And regardless of your doctor or his office, the infertility workup is actually a work*out*. It requires commitment, perseverance, and patience. Being childless against our will is stressful. Avoid targeting your doctor for any frustration or anger you may feel for your childless state.

If you have a physician who is helping you through infertility, work at being appreciative. Be grateful you even have access to that doctor and to technology. Just thirty years ago childless couples did not *have* the options out there today. And, as previously mentioned, there are few couples who have the finances to even consider a medical resolution for infertility. It's easy to forget some of our trials (navigating the difficulties of medical care) are blessings in disguise.

INFORMATION V. EDUCATION

Some well-meaning people will offer advice which is medically off-base. There's also information regarding infertility we may read or hear about which *seems* logical but is incorrect or outdated. Should you choose to conduct research on your own, I recommend you work to obtain information from a reliable and reputable source which is keeping current with or leading the charge on medical technology.

Mankind is only as knowledgeable as God permits, and even medical geniuses are prone to taking views that are not grounded in God's revealed truth. It is my prayer you will take purposeful measures to ensure you don't substitute the wisdom of man for the wisdom of God.

GOD—THE "ABSOLUTE RESOURCE"

God transcends every resource man can unearth. He is greater than the best wellspring of advice we can discover. He is more powerful than the finest physician money can retain. God and God alone is the One Who is able to open and close the womb no matter what we may choose to believe or what credit people may try to take. It's God who provides us with increased knowledge in regard to causes for infertility and ways to combat it, and *nothing* changes the fact that it is God who creates new life. Both the Old and the New Testament speak to the fact it is God who is the giver of children. *We are still living "in Bible times" and God is fully able to perform any type of miracle in the lives of ordinary people He chooses.*

When the angel Gabriel appeared to Mary and told her she would bear a son who would be called the Son of the Most High, and the Lord God would give Him the throne of His father David, she knew enough about "how babies were made" to inquire as to how this would come about since she was a virgin. Gabriel responded to her question with specifics and ended by stating "And behold, even your relative Elizabeth has also conceived a son in her old age; and she who was called barren is now in her sixth month. For nothing will be impossible with God" (Luke 1:36-37).

In Psalm 127:3 we're told "Behold, children are a gift of the Lord; the fruit of the womb is a reward." And I love Psalm 113:5-9, which says:

> Who is like the LORD our God,
> Who is enthroned on high,
> Who humbles Himself to behold
> The things that are in heaven and in the earth?
> He raises the poor from the dust,
> And lifts the needy from the ash heap,
> To make them sit with princes,
> With the princes of his people.
> He makes the barren woman abide in the house
> As a joyful mother of children.
> Praise the LORD!

God *is* your greatest resource, dear sister, whether you are rolling in money or wondering how you'll put together the next meal.

We serve a God who is the very Author of Life. I know of several couples who were told by physicians they would never be able to conceive, and God proved those intelligent professionals wrong. My sweet friend, if you're a part of the majority who does *not* have the option of going to a specialist and using medical technology to achieve pregnancy or receive treatment to help prevent miscarriages, you are no less eligible in God's economy to give birth to a healthy baby than anyone else. Alternatively, if you are one who has been through the infertility work*out* with all medical technology failing to help you, you also are no less eligible in God's mercy to give birth to a healthy baby than anyone else.

We may not want to look at truth so openly, but the opposite is also true: If God has determined for reasons known to Him and unknown to us (other than that His faithfulness never falls short), He may close fast our wombs and no amount of technology, prayer, or faith will open them. This is another reason why every chapter in this book is important to read and prayerfully ponder. It takes a journey of time and faith to truly understand and accept the fact that God is doing what is best for us; *second best is an unknown to Him.* May we take full refuge in that truth and hold fast to His Word.

I know that You can do all things, and that no purpose of Yours can be thwarted. Job 42:2.

MY PRAYER FOR YOU: I marvel at how You invite and instruct us to call You our Father. You are the Mastermind and Creator of family and the giver of life. I humbly ask, Father, that You will open the wombs of us, Your adopted daughters, as You see fit. May nothing about pursuing pregnancy distract from this beloved reader's understanding that You are above all and that her heart can safely trust in You.

14

You and Your Husband

WHEN GOD ANSWERED MY PLEA to minister to women who were struggling through infertility, He had you *and* your husband in mind. I was overwhelmed and thinking about you. God was perfectly in control and thinking about you and your spouse.

Although infertility can bring a couple closer together, it more frequently causes a strain. Any difficulty or pain we encounter as an individual or a couple can cause us to take our eyes off Christ and demand our full attention. A perfect example of this is when we accidentally slam our finger in a drawer. The damaged tissues and nerve endings immediately send signals from the finger to the brain. The brain then sends out the message: "Your finger is hurt! Your finger is hurt!" in order to immediately facilitate the removal of your finger from the source of its pain. While our brains are sending out the urgent message "Your finger is hurt! Your finger is hurt!" none of us simultaneously think: *I love and trust God so much. And I wonder if my man is having a good day?*

And nobody needs to tell you the pain of infertility is much tougher to deal with than slamming one's finger in a drawer.

~

That enemy of old is out there. Although the Bible tells us Satan can make himself appear as if he were an angel of light (see 2 Corinthians 11:13-14), let's imagine him appearing as evil as he really is (see John 8:44). Try to picture him now, crouching in the cover of tall grasses and scrubland with his wicked eyes fastened on a target we're unable to see. Straining at the ends of their leashes, which he's holding in a sinewy hand, are tigers. You suddenly realize they are Satan's tigers of falsehood we met earlier. With his free hand Satan touches the tigers one at a time to let them know they will soon be released. They're sleek and muscular with sharp teeth that have tasted the flesh of men and women before.

The object of Satan's attention steps into view, and you realize with alarm it's your husband. At that moment, with evil delight, Satan unleashes the first tiger of falsehood. It springs into action! The moment the tiger's claws find their mark the second tiger is released. This one, too, races through the underbrush fueled by the lust for blood. Your spouse, with one tiger on him, is still on his feet, valiantly trying to fight the beast off. The second tiger strikes low, grabbing your husband's leg with its powerful claws and sinking its teeth deep into his calf muscle. Then the third tiger is unleashed and moves like a bullet. Satan howls in ecstasy as the frenzied tigers of falsehood proceed to rip and tear him apart with accusations:

※ Look at your wife, Loser. You can't even make her happy!

✳ Real men don't feel this kind of pain.

✳ You haven't figured out marriage yet; how do you think you could possibly manage parenting?

✳ She only wants intimacy with you in the hopes of getting pregnant.

✳ God is punishing you!

✳ Maybe you married the wrong woman.

✳ Suffer in silence, Buddy. You can't afford to let yourself be vulnerable.

Just as you and I sometimes smile and appear to be fine on the outside when we're really suffering on the inside, so does your husband. He may be wrestling with tigers of falsehood with or without your knowledge. Unless we wives learn to be more observant and ask better questions, we may not know how our husbands are struggling or thinking. We need to recognize they need our love and support more than we realize or they may be letting us know.

Perhaps you're thinking, "Wow! If she only *knew* what I am living with!" Your husband may be making your life miserable with his dissatisfaction over being childless. He may be reacting to his pain by inflicting pain on you, pushing you hard to "find out whatever's wrong with you." Maybe your husband isn't a believer in Christ (yet). If such is the case—whether he's a sweet guy or a huge challenge—his spiritual needs are urgent. Whatever descriptive phrases come to your mind when thinking about your husband, this chapter is wholly applicable to your situation.

In chapter 4 we asked ourselves what falsehoods Satan has unleashed at us. Now is the time to get out paper and pen or pencil and settle into a comfortable spot, if you are able. There are a few questions below for you to ponder in relation to your husband. With soul searching and prayer, please answer them honestly and write down your answers.

1. What tigers of falsehood can you identify which have been unleashed on your husband by Satan?

2. What are some falsehoods he might be struggling with that you haven't stopped to think about before?

3. What are some possible falsehoods you may have grown accustomed to believe about your husband? Your marriage?

The next question involves a possible need for repentance on your part. Let's first pause to consider what repentance is and isn't.

It's all too easy in a marriage to say, "I'm sorry" and think we've done our duty. Yet repenting is *not* saying, "I made a mistake" or "I'm sorry I did that." True repentance is to admit we have sinned. We recognize that we chose to do the opposite of what God has shown to be the right action. However, there's far more involved in repenting than mere recognition of our wrongdoing. Repentance involves our agreement with God we have sinned and we inwardly—and perhaps outwardly—grieve for having done so; we must then methodically and deliberately change course (direction). Repentance is getting *off* the wrong path and getting *onto* the right one. This means that in the matter over which we are repenting, it's our heart's desire to *never* commit that sin again. Repentance also demands we humble ourselves and ask the person we have wronged, if living and accessible, to forgive us, specifically naming how we have wronged them. We should do this with God before we engage anyone else in the process.

With that little refresher in mind, you should be ready to resume thinking about your husband and marriage, and writing down your answers:

4. Have there been any falsehoods unleashed at your husband by *you*? If so, what are they? And, if so, are you willing to repent for what you have done?

5. Are you willing to forgive your husband for any emotional hurt he may have caused you and be willing to work with him at restoration? Are you willing to forgive him even if he shows no sign of repentance?

If the teamwork and communication in your marriage has deteriorated to the point where you're unable as a couple to discuss deeper issues, I encourage you to pray about the need for a change and seek out sound counsel as a couple. Assistance may come in the form of a godly Christian couple in your support structure or through a *solid* Bible-based Christian counselor. If your husband is unwilling to meet with anyone, I encourage you to pray the same way and seek out sound counsel for yourself. Remember, however, there is no substitute for God's wisdom found in His Word.

I recognize these aren't easy matters to deal with. And even though you and I may have never met, God has given me a deep and sincere love for you. So please accept this: I love you. And please hang in here with me.

Despite what may be our own pain, we as wives need to pro-actively seek ways in which to minister to and encourage our husbands. Work to make the man you married feel like more than your personal, walking sperm donor. Perhaps your husband needs to be affirmed for who he is rather than what he can produce. Explore the depths of his mind; cook his favorite meal; ask God to show you how to please him. There are many ways we can communicate with our husbands and not all of them are verbal. You need to let him know you love him and are crazy about him. Frankly, our husbands need to know they will be enough for us should our plans and dreams of parenthood never come to fruition.

If we're struggling to love our husbands and are *not* crazy about them, we should be encouraged to know God can teach us how to love them:

> Older women likewise are to be reverent in their behavior, not malicious gossips, nor enslaved to much wine, teaching what is good, that they may encourage the young women to love their husbands, to love their children, to be sensible, pure, workers at home, kind, being subject to their own husbands, that the word of God may not be dishonored. (Titus 2:3-5)

Despite what movies we have watched or what we grew up hoping for, the Bible shows us that falling in love does *not* just happen. According to the book of Titus, the older women in Christ's church are to be teaching the younger women to *love their husbands*. It should come as no surprise to us that God recognizes our husbands aren't so wonderful as to guarantee our undying love and devotion. We have to be taught to love them. And it's very interesting to observe we're to be taught to love our husbands before being taught to love our children. Hmm, husbands come first! And loving them is a choice; a command from the very heart of God.

Likewise, God calls husbands to love their wives as Christ loved His church, with a sacrificial love. (Oh, my!) As wives, we're not to be taught to love our husbands *if* they love us the way they're supposed to. We're simply to be taught to love them. We are to choose to love them and learn how to love them. In other words, we're to be intentional and proactive in our love for our husbands.

⁂

There's an equine training principle which actually serves as an excellent example regarding this need. It goes like this: *The strongest halter in the world is the horse's mind.*

A halter is a man-made product which slides or buckles onto a horse's head, enabling a handler to lead the horse around and tie it to posts. If we're able to get a horse to *think* it wants to follow us where we want it to go or stand quietly where we want it to stand, it really doesn't matter whether the horse is wearing a halter made of leather, rope, or pigeon feathers—or if it's wearing a halter at all. It's the *mind* which causes the horse to willingly follow us or stand quietly where we want it to stand. Similarly, the best way for us to learn (or relearn) how to love our husbands is by permitting God's Word to reprogram our thinking about our husbands and our marriages. If our minds and hearts are engaged in loving our husbands, we're then able to become intentional and proactive in loving them well.

Although I can't help but wish I embraced this process earlier in my own marriage, I humbly offer for your consideration a number of avenues in which we can more intentionally and proactively love our husbands:

THROUGH PRAYER

Specific, consistent time in prayer on our husband's behalf should be a part of our daily life. A few good ways in which to pray for him are that he will:

✳ Have or come to have a love for truth and be in God's Word on a consistent basis

✳ Respond to God's Word in humility and joy

✳ Love or come to love God with his whole heart

✳ Have good Christian men as friends and mentors

✳ Recognize God's blessings in his life

✳ Grow in the knowledge and grace of the Lord Jesus Christ

✳ Know God's gift of grace and forgiveness

✳ Be blessed by God with discernment and wisdom

✳ Be pure and purified in his daily walk

Being a good observer and listener will help you know in which areas your man could use extra prayer support. Let him know regularly that you love him and are praying for him, asking if there are any specific needs you can be praying about. If he's cranky or easily annoyed over spiritual matters, it isn't necessary to tell him how you are praying. Continue steadfast in prayer on his behalf, however, and shower him with respect and kindness at every opportunity God gives you.

THROUGH GOAL SETTING

These are goals we set for ourselves about our husbands, not goals *we* want our *husbands* to have. (Sorry, my friend!) If you'll recall our discussion in chapter 9 about The Worthy Goal, you likely picked up on the fact we should have personal goals relating to our husbands. What needs does your husband have, and how can you help meet them? Like all of us, he has a definite need for prayer. So prayer on his behalf is a very specific goal you can write down, laying out how often you will strive to pray for him each day. Our husbands have physical needs, emotional needs, and spiritual needs. We should develop specific steps for *us* to take to help meet each area of need. Does he need a cleaner home atmosphere than you've been providing? If so, write down specific daily, weekly, and monthly goals for yourself as to how you can improve your home's atmosphere. Does he need you to listen to his frustrations without you telling him how to solve his problems? Then make yourself goals specific to that need. One of the challenges is to not set goals for how you want your husband to be, but what he needs from *you*, his wife. Our goals are about controlling ourselves, not others! If we set goals to be in God's Word regularly, for example, it's one way of loving our husbands. Our spiritual growth is, or will become, a gift to him.

BY DEEPENING OUR LEARNING

We should be taking advantage of tools to learn more about our husbands. One of these may be to develop the art of asking questions designed to engage him in better quality communication. For example, you may want to consider telling him about your thoughts as you read through the chapter on the

Lonely Path and ask him what, if anything, has ever made him feel he was on a Lonely Path? If you have a godly woman in your life who appears to have wisdom and a healthy marriage, ask her for ideas as to how you can deepen your understanding about your husband and daily demonstrate love to him in a practical manner. In addition to the Bible, carefully select books to read by spiritually wise individuals on marriage and apply principles which will change your heart and actions to your husband's betterment.

The above principles of loving our husbands deeply will be invaluable to our marriages *and* to our children, should God grant us our petitions of Him for a child. Can you imagine having a strategic, pro-active plan to pray for your husband and child every day, setting goals for yourself to help meet their needs, and to deepen your learning about the way God made them as you are being encouraged to do today for your husband? Wow!

"The Love Chapter"

If I speak with the tongues of men and of angels, but do not have love, I have become a noisy gong or a clanging cymbal. And if I have the gift of prophecy, and know all mysteries and all knowledge; and if I have all faith, so as to move mountains, but do not have love, I am nothing. And if I give all my possessions to feed the poor, and if I deliver my body to be burned, but do not have love, it profits me nothing.

Love is patient; love is kind, and is not jealous; love does not brag and is not arrogant, does not act unbecomingly; it does not seek its own, is not provoked, does not take into account a wrong suffered, does not rejoice in unrighteousness, but rejoices with the truth; bears all things, believes all things, hopes all things, endures all things.

Love never fails; but if there are gifts of prophecy, they will be done away; if there are tongues, they will cease; if there is knowledge, it will be done away. For we know in part, and we prophesy in part; but when the perfect comes, the partial will be done away.

When I was a child, I used to speak as a child, think as a child, reason as a child; when I became a man, I did away with childish things. For now we see in a mirror dimly, but then face to face; now I know in part, but then I shall know fully just as I also have been fully known.

But now abide faith, hope, love, these three; but the greatest of these is love.

—1 Corinthians 13

When you're intentional in your communication and love, even in times of your own pain, *you* can be used by God to help encourage and build up this man you are hoping to have a child with. Should God grant us our desires to become mothers, we will need to be equipped with the tools to love and serve others unconditionally—no matter what hurts or concerns we may be carrying, or whether or not those we live with are responding in ways which are God's ways.

❧

MY PRAYER FOR YOU: My Precious Lord, I know breathtaking hope must include loving exhortation. You have a way of moving us out of our comfort zones. You invade areas of our minds and hearts we don't even want to have to think about. But, Lord God, I ask that You will bless this one for continuing to journey through this book, and I earnestly pray You will reveal to her not only Your great love for her, but of Your great love for her husband. May she partner with You and seek Your face to love him in accordance with Your Word. Use that resurrection power to make her marriage strong and her husband the type of leader only You can make him be for Your glory and our joy. Amen.

15

Is Adoption An Option?

FEWER PEOPLE HAVE RESISTED adoption any harder than *me*. Does that surprise you?

Many times in my anguish over not having children, Brad would gently encourage me by stating perhaps it was God's desire for us to adopt. I should say while Brad *attempted* to encourage me to consider adoption; his suggestions and tenderness were often met with heat and a fresh flow of tears.

It didn't seem to matter we had friends and acquaintances who had adopted darling kids and were delighted with how things worked out for them. I resented the thought of *us* adopting. Brad, who is wonderfully persuasive with me, had no success in changing my mind despite his patient endeavors. I just refused to go there.

How could a person be growing and learning so much in one area of trust in God for a family yet obstinately dig in her heels and rebel at another? I was uncertain at the time, but that's right where I was: in open rebellion against adoption. I found myself beginning to dislike the word. Why should I have to even *hear* it, I wondered?

"Lord," I reasoned. "I want to be pregnant and You can easily make it happen! I'd like to see Brad's characteristics in our kids. I'd like know what it feels like to have our son or daughter growing and moving in my womb."

It was also disheartening to learn the costs of a typical adoption would likely be a financial impossibility for us. Why should we have to endure hardship in so many areas, I asked myself, while having to settle for what I viewed as a second-best option? It just didn't seem fair.

My close-mindedness towards adopting a baby lasted for almost a year. I was miserable, yet somewhat content to stay resolute. One day, however, Brad surprised me.

After yet another tearful wave of depression, Brad looked at me unsympathetically and shared how he had been praying for over *half a year* that I would become reasonable and open to adopting. He said that he, too, was anxious to become a parent and precious time was slipping by. Although he never raised his voice, he bluntly told me he believed we should sign up for adoption and that he expected me to back him up on it. My shock was complete when Brad instructed, "I want you to call Dallas first thing tomorrow morning. Get the name and telephone number of the adoption agency they used and call it to get started on whatever needs to happen to get an adoption underway."

Over the years we had always been able to work out disagreements quickly and with minimal damage. But we had hit an impasse over adoption. Brad recognized we were like a couple sitting at the side of the road with a flat tire, and one of us wasn't permitting the other to fix it. He was ready to change the tire, so to speak, and wanted me to hand him the jack. Not unreasonable.

That broke me. Unless I wanted to fling away the values our marriage was based on, I needed to get back to thinking about my husband's desires and not just my own. It was also disturbing to face the fact that I'd been holding *Brad* up on his own dreams and pursuits of parenthood. What a hypocrite I was to be caring and praying for women who were suffering through childlessness while failing to meaningfully consider my own husband's pain! My insensitivity to Brad was a sin I had to confess and repent of before God and then seek forgiveness from Brad on.

⋇

The following morning, with immense dread, I picked up the phone and called my friend Dallas. Minutes later, I was dialing the number she had given me for the adoption agency with cold, trembling fingers.

Why was I shaking? I wondered.

I realized there was, amazingly, an *excitement* building up in me I didn't understand. By the time the receptionist's voice came on the line, a wild, joyful pounding had taken over my heart and I felt like shouting, "Hi! I want to adopt a baby! Oh, I *want* to adopt a baby!"

Brad, somewhat apprehensively, called me later in the morning to see how I was doing. He wasn't mentally prepared when I excitedly told him about the possibility of adopting. And two days later, when seated at our kitchen table filling out a questionnaire from the adoption agency, he blinked at his previously resistant wife who was saying, "This is so wonderful, honey! This could be our only chance of having a brown-eyed child!"

I am sure Brad was wondering: *What on earth has happened to her? Is this the same person I couldn't persuade to adopt?*

⁂

I marveled at the change. At the time, I was unable to understand what had happened to me. Yet later, I realized God used Brad to help me overcome a *tremendous* hurdle—my death grip on the feelings I *had* to conceive, carry, and deliver our children or I would not ever be a *real* mom. A few months later, while we were pursuing both adoption and nearly going broke seeing the infertility specialist, God led me to a point where He asked even more of me.

Was I willing to be childless if, for some reason, God firmly closed the door on pregnancy and adoption? How far did my willingness and trust in Him go?

⁂

When I least expected it, God was asking me to face the "Big Fear." Do you recall my having shared a subconscious worry that giving in to God "too radically" would have disastrous results? *What was God doing*, I wondered? Here I had finally come to a point of being willing to adopt, and now, in His quiet way, God was asking me to be willing to let go of *that* too?

Oh, God, my Father. Please, no! My heart cried. Immediately, His Holy Spirit put these words in my mind:

Do you love Me, child, more than anything?
Are you willing to put all your dreams and
aspirations of being a parent on the altar?
Do you trust Me enough?

Like our father of the faith, Abraham, it seemed as if God were asking me to climb the mountain, build an altar, and slay something most precious to me (see Genesis 22:1-2). I was facing a spiritual battle within my own heart.

The weapons of our warfare are not of the flesh, but divinely powerful for the destruction of fortresses. We are destroying speculations and every lofty thing raised up against the knowledge of God, and we are taking every thought to the obedience of Christ. (2 Corinthians 10:4-5).

It was then I recognized my dream of parenthood *had* been raised up against the knowledge of God, for I was wondering, indirectly, *Is God worthy of my trust in this area?* God, who intimately desires to purify us, knew fully what was high and lifted up in my heart. He then asked me to destroy that fortress, to bring my thoughts captive into the very same sphere as Christ's obedience to God the Father. My high and lofty fortress was my dream and desire of becoming a mother. God was asking me to offer it up to Him… as a sacrifice.

※

Abraham, when commanded by God, was willing to sacrifice his only son, the promised heir, when it surely seemed senseless for him to do so. Yet through many years, trials, and painful lessons, Abraham—by this time an old man—had learned God was worthy of his trust *regardless* of what God required of him or commanded him to do (see Genesis 22:3-6).

At the last moment possible, God sent an angel to stop Abraham from thrusting the knife blade into his son's body (see Genesis 22:7-11). And Abraham didn't argue!

❧

We may ask why God orchestrated this stressful exercise in mankind's history. Do you think He wanted to watch Abraham and Isaac squirm? Do you think God derived some sick pleasure from asking Abraham to do the hardest thing in the world for him?

No. It would be contrary to God's nature (see Ephesians 2:4-5).

Is it possible God felt insecure and needed Abraham to prove he loved Him more than he loved Isaac?

No. God has no insecurities, and He is all-knowing! (see Psalm 147:5). He alone knows man's heart (see Psalm 44:21).

The answer for this astonishing and mysterious occurrence lies in the Bible's clarity of God the Father, God the Son, and God the Holy Spirit having always had a plan for mankind to be the beneficiaries of a Savior—a flawless sacrifice—which would permit believing, grateful people to be forgiven of their sins and enter into a marvelous, personal relationship with Him (the "Three in One"). It was *never* God's plan to have Abraham physically sacrifice his long-awaited-for son, because Isaac was not perfect nor was he the Son of God; Isaac, therefore, was not a suitable sacrifice to accomplish the finished work necessary for salvation. It had always been God's plan to give *His* only son, Jesus Christ, as that spotless, holy, necessary sacrifice for our sins.

Abraham built the altar and laid upon it his beloved son. It was a clear demonstration of just how much he trusted in his *God*. While Abraham was in the process of exercising radical faith in God, little did he know God would rock the world with a clear, unmistakable marker to point us to the coming Messiah, who was the sacrifice God did *not* "replace" or withhold (see John 3:16).

Did putting *my* dreams of parenthood on the altar mean they would never be realized? I didn't know!

There is no account of Abraham weeping at the altar he built under his son's watchful gaze. Scripture tells us Abraham communicated beforehand to his servants both he *and* his son would return after they went on the mountain to worship God. He knew God would either provide a substitute sacrifice or raise his son back from the dead.

I believe Abraham built a *spiritual* altar in his heart and sacrificed his most cherished human dreams and possessions on it before he ever built the *physical* one. With less faith than Abraham, I built my spiritual altar and wept in the process. But I meant every word.

This hurts, God, but I'm sincere. For You to do with as You please, here I sacrifice what has been high and lifted up in my heart.

❧

Through the trials and testing of infertility, God has taught me to completely trust his Word, and to obey it regardless of the circumstances. This is a valuable lesson I long for you to possess, for it is critical for us to fully surrender everything to

Christ in order to live a life of joy and freedom, free from fear and anxiety.

In time, I learned to trust God through infertility. That experience served me well as we took steps to adopt. Also, having put the entire baby issue on the altar helped me in ways I cannot express when facing a whole new set of fears and apprehensions about adoption:

> Will we even qualify for adoption or be selected by a birth mother after having sold our nice home and moved into an ugly four-plex in the middle of nowhere? All because we decided to make sacrifices to support a new Christian ministry we believed in?
>
> Where will the money come from to pull this off?
>
> Will our adopted baby be healthy?
>
> Will we sensibly handle ignorant or rude questions and comments from others when they learn our child is adopted?
>
> Will the child feel rejected if and when learning about having been placed for adoption?
>
> If our adopted child searches for and finds his birth mother, will his love for her surpass his love for me?
>
> What if our adopted baby is really ugly? Or slow? Or non-athletic? Will I blame the biological parents and have resentment?
>
> Can the birth mother change her mind and take the baby away from us?
>
> If we adopt and then get pregnant later, will I love the children the same?

Will we have the needed support and understanding
from others if we adopt?

The decision to pursue adoption should never be marginalized. But don't let your fears or any criticism from others deter you from prayerful consideration of it as a means to have one or more children.

I realized my questions and fears about adoption closely mirrored those which had tormented me in the past when I was unable to conceive. Questions such as:

* ❋ Will I ever have a baby?
* ❋ Is something wrong with me?
* ❋ Doesn't God care?
* ❋ Why me?

God helped me through the mire of them all, and although Satan did his best to cause me great fear and anxiety about adoption, he was defeated. By God's grace, I had built my altar! I had turned over to God the babies I dreamed of. And God, praise His name, blessed me with peace.

When a question or fear about adoption ran through my mind, I deliberately moved it aside saying, "It doesn't matter. God is in control. I rest in Your wisdom and power, dear Lord."

Only God and His Word can give that kind of assurance.

This is steadfast hope—trust.

I began to realize such trust in God for everything would help me throughout my life. Perhaps after becoming a parent, I might face a whole new set of fears: fears about my child needing emergency surgery or his or her safety at school. Regardless of becoming a parent, there are other uncertainties in life. I could discover I have cancer, my husband could lose his job, our home could burn to the ground, or God *could* call us to a jungle as missionaries where snakes and boiled rats become my experience!

What am I attempting to emphasize? Simply this: No matter what, we *will* face countless opportunities to be anxious, afraid, bitter, or worried throughout our lives. Are you learning to obey God's Word *now* in a practical way through infertility? If so, you will be better equipped to face the uncertainties of adoption, or any other difficulties you encounter.

At this point in time, do you even consider adoption an alternative? If so, you likely have numerous questions and concerns—which is normal. If you do have a bag full of questions in one hand, see to it you're holding fast to God's Word in the other. With each new set of questions and fears, hand them over to God and cling all the more to your Bible and God's promises. Secondarily, as a couple, you may also want to consider receiving counsel and encouragement through a Christian adoption agency, support group, or counselor about legitimate concerns you have.

James instructs us, "If any of you lacks wisdom, let him ask of God who gives to all men generously and without reproach, and it will be given to him" (James 1:5).

If you and your husband have been trying to have children without success, you may want to seriously consider signing up for adoption *now*. There is no set waiting period; the time before placement of a baby varies with adoption agencies, availability of babies, and other factors. I have heard of couples waiting for five or six years, and others who had a baby in a year. There are some who have only a few months to wait. My point is this: you have little to lose by starting the adoption process immediately.

⁂

Can something go wrong? Yes, absolutely—from a *worldly* perspective. A private adoption may get underway and fall through, and some couples have experienced this heart-breaking scenario more than once. The grief is comparable to going to great lengths to become pregnant only to lose the baby through miscarriage or stillbirth. These are almost *unthinkable* trials, and we may wonder where God is in the midst of them. To believe we're following God's leading and then experience indescribable pain can rip our faith apart, which is certainly what our enemy wants. Yet it doesn't mean God isn't with us when we're going through it, or He isn't orchestrating something beautiful out of tragedy (which we may not see until we reach heaven). Adoption most certainly carries its own set of risks; however, when we stop and think about it, the entire act of parenting is beset with risks.

If you take steps to adopt and happen to conceive and safely carry a baby to term while waiting for placement, you may need to drop out of the process (a requirement with some adoption agencies). Yet if no progress is made on having your children biologically, you'll be just that much closer to adopting your children, and *that* is thrilling too!

⁂

It was God Almighty who masterminded adoption when He made a way for *us* to become *His* children (see Galatians 4:4-5). No human being is born without a nature bent towards sinning (see Romans 3:23). To think a perfect, holy God would want to make a way for us to come to Him, live with Him, and be fully identified with Him—*adopted* by Him—is truly incomprehensible. Through Christ's sacrificial death on the cross of Calvary, and His burial and resurrection three days later, He paid the sin debt and God declares worthy all who believe in His Son (see Romans 10:9). We then become *heirs of Christ*, adopted into God's family, in which everything God has is ours!

> For you have not received a spirit of slavery leading to
> fear again, but you have received a spirit of adoption
> as sons by which we cry out, "Abba! Father!" The Spirit
> Himself testifies with our spirit that we are children of
> God, and if children, heirs also, heirs of God and fellow
> heirs with Christ. (Romans 8:15-17)

This redirects my thinking. In our own personal pursuit of parenthood, I have thought most often about myself: what I desire as a parent and what my dreams of parenthood entail. When I look deeper at God's miraculous adoption of *me*—a defective, failure-prone human being—my spirit quiets in humble awe and gratitude. And then… you guessed it. I begin struggling to breathe at the wonder of it.

Are you with me at the picnic table?

Adoption is a beautiful act, and most adoptive parents I know feel couples who have not added to their family in this way have missed a wonderful experience.

Should you find yourself wistfully observing mothers running errands with their children, playing with their kids in the park, or making the school run, please remember: you may be looking at the blessed results of one or more adoptions.

Whether or not you consider adoption as an option for becoming parents, will you pause with me this moment and earnestly thank God for wanting us? For pursuing us? For being willing to adopt us?

❧

MY PRAYER FOR YOU: Dear Lord, I first of all praise and thank You. Thank You for the amazing gift of Your Son as our substitute/sacrifice. Thank You for Your willingness to adopt us into a perfect, forever family. I ask You to please bless this reader with gratitude and provide the healing and direction she and her husband need regarding children. I pray You will bless them with unity as a couple and help them to offer up in sacrifice anything that may be elevated in their hearts and minds above You; for their good and Your glory.

16

Miscarriage: Your Unforgettable Due Date(s)

PERHAPS YOU'VE SUFFERED a miscarriage and tried briefly explaining to a friend or family member how painful it was for you. If so, I want you to know I'm so sorry. And I shudder to think this naive question may have come your way: "But when it's in the first trimester, isn't it just like having a regular period?"

You may have braved the storm and shared your honest thought-reaction to their question. Then again, the thoughts may have just seared their way through your soul.

Just like a period? No!

A menstrual cycle is a menstrual cycle. A miscarriage is a death!

*Menstrual cycle tissues are just that. A miscarriage is…
well, our baby, our dream. Our plans now gone. We won't
ever be able to hold our growing child (was it a boy or a
girl?) in our arms or laugh with him or her. I will be strong,
but you must let me grieve!*

*Just like a period!? How could it be? A part of me has died,
never to be replaced!*

This chapter, among others, is one I never knew I would be
writing for you.

⚜

After opening up about our infertility, God began to bring
women into my life, one by one, who needed help in the cru-
cible of childlessness. This informal ministry eventually caused
me to cross paths with women who had conceived and lost
their unborn children. I ached for those who had miscarriages.
How could they possibly endure the emotional and spiritual pain,
I wondered? Would my strong convictions about trusting God
hold true for them? Would they find God's Word to be of last-
ing encouragement? And what if it happened to me? Could I
bear up under such agony?

This special chapter, in a way, is a miracle. God had a perfect
plan and timing, and experiences for me to live out I never saw
coming. Early on, He permitted me to experience the pain and
anxiety of being childless against my will. God then sustained
me through the frightening process of adoption. He later
blessed us with a pregnancy that ended in miscarriage.

I hadn't wanted you to know that. This chapter was origi-
nally written in the hope of ministering to others without my

having to personally experience the death of a baby. As time went on and God firmly showed Himself to be unhurried in revealing to me how and when He would permit me to finish this book, I rewrote this chapter with much deeper emotion and understanding. Yet I still petitioned God to help me to do so without sharing with you the full depths of my experience. My concern? I wanted you to hear less about me and more about God. I was afraid if you read about any more miracles He performed in my life, you might become discouraged rather than encouraged. But God gently reminded me this was His chapter, His book, and His ministry to you, and I actually had very little to do with it.

If you've had one or more miscarriages, my prayer is you will recognize God is fully aware of your pain. He is present with you when questions come from other people, and when you have questions from within your own heart. He's not only *aware* and *present*, but He's hurting with you.

In the following section, I address some painful questions or comments you might have heard if you've experienced a miscarriage. Usually these are spoken by well-meaning individuals who just have no idea how insensitive their words might be.

"Did you do something to cause the miscarriage?"

This question occasionally slips out before people stop to think about the additional grief it could bring. What woman doesn't somehow blame herself for her miscarriage—at least momentarily—whether rational or not?

I should have seen that patch of ice. To think I was so careless as to fall!

Did the medication that said it was okay to take during pregnancy bring this on?

Was the work or exercise I did that day too strenuous?

Was I not forgiven for the abortion(s)?

Would things have been different had I been in better physical condition before conceiving?

There are numerous threads of pain, anguish, fear, and remorse surrounding miscarriage. And the *term itself* can even be disheartening; it can feel to the woman as though she somehow failed to do an acceptable job of harboring the life within her womb. Just look at other ways the prefix *mis* is used:

"*Mis*calculation" (you calculated wrong)
"*Mis*take" (you didn't choose the right option)
"*Mis*managed" (you managed poorly)
"*Mis*carriage" (you failed to carry your baby to term)

There really isn't an adequate word to accompany something as awful as the loss of an unborn child. Yet the term mis*carriage* doesn't do anything to ease the pain of the wounded.

"It's nature's way of handling babies with severe health problems. It's probably a good thing it happened even though going through it is rough."

Sometimes, if we are attuned to God, He gives us a peace that is hard to put into words regardless of what caused the miscarriage. It's a peace that is unnatural—supernatural. Yet who would have thought peace and pain—such pain!—could abide within the same vessel, at the very same time? And why assume we wouldn't love and delight in a child with health problems? This was a little person—our baby!

"God will give you other children. At least you know you can get pregnant."

Will God give us other children? Will I conceive again? And if I do, will it be a successful pregnancy? I don't know all of God's intricate workings, although I trust Him. He will do what is best. But He may not give us another child and, even if He does, I grieve the loss of this child, this life, my lost little one. Saying goodbye is so hard when there wasn't a chance to really say hello!

Those of us who suffer from miscarriage are briefly pitied, perhaps encouraged, and then to a degree expected to bounce back almost as if nothing had happened. While it's true we must carry on, many people don't stop to consider that the couple who loses an unborn child has lost a family member, just as surely as the couple whose toddler or grade-schooler has died. The toddler's parents weep over memories and lost dreams as they painfully sift through their deceased child's clothes and toys. Those of us who have miscarried may weep over the sorting of maternity clothes no longer needed, baby shoes which may never cradle a foot, the trauma of delivering a stillborn baby, and/or dreams which were abruptly and unexpectedly terminated.

The funeral for the child everyone knew who was taken in death draws our attention to the grieving family. The hearse, casket, and flowers shout: *This family has lost their child!* We know they will never be quite the same. We recognize the vacant place brought on by death can never really be filled by another. Where we once saw a family of perhaps four or five, one is now glaringly missing. They were named and known. There's one less plate at the table; one less person in the "family row" at church; one less seatbelt to be buckled.

Your friends or family members who've never themselves experienced a miscarriage are often unable to fully grasp what has happened to you. There was no funeral. No casket. No fewer plates at your breakfast table. If you miscarried early in the pregnancy, you may even *look* the same as you did before.

But in the quiet of your home, the quiet of your heart, your life has been dramatically altered. Prying eyes may never see the unexpected hurts or scars you bear from the loss of your unborn baby (or, for some of you, the loss of your *babies*).

It is a time when God alone can soothe those deepest hurts and heal our hearts. It's a time God can—and will—restore our souls, if we let Him.

Yet, even when we *do* experience God's peace and healing through miscarriage, there are times when the pangs still hit us. Times that, when it's all said and done, are just plain *hard*.

Like the due date.

❧

You learned of your baby's conception. How fun! What a joy! Your doctor probably smiled when announcing your little one's expected arrival date. The good news about your pregnancy spread. The hottest question became: "What's the due date?" It likely wasn't long before you didn't even have to think about it. That date undoubtedly rolled off your tongue like beautiful music. No matter that only about 5 percent of the babies born ever hit their actual due date, the date became chiseled in your mind. It had become a special day in a suddenly special year. *Your baby's anticipated arrival date!*

The miscarriage occurs. You agonize at the loss, despair over the emptiness, and wade through the grief. In time, you may "get on with life." Healing (hopefully) takes place, but there's something still hanging out there. And you won't be able to forget it: The due date.

That special day on the calendar that now seems to mock you.

The point in time earmarked for one of the most special occurrences in your life. The womb is now empty, but the date is not forgotten.

❧

Being aware of the looming date might be expected in individuals who nursed bitterness or self-pity, but for the woman who has truly experienced God's healing through such a loss, it *can* be a bit surprising.

Yet from the time you learned new life was forming within your framework, you began changing as a person. Thoughts and priorities changed. You had someone *else* to think about, eat for, and plan for. Your world suddenly enlarged. You thought of possible names; you perhaps even settled on one. Losing your unborn baby will never alter the fact that you became a mother.

We think of Mother's Day cards and celebrations for those mothers whose children we see or know. Nonetheless, you were a little one's mother. Death doesn't change that. Your mother's instinct and heart were already fully engaged and operating.

It is the mother's heart which remembers a date on the calendar others soon forget.

❧

God assured Brad and me of His love during and following the loss of our unborn baby. Despite that, I feared I might think of God as unloving or myself as a defective Christian as my due date approached. As if we don't have enough unhealthy thoughts of our own to wrestle with, Satan is all too happy to provide us with even more, and I knew this. I recognized he would be remembering our baby's due date, too. His goal would be to reopen old wounds and sever our walk with God. He looks for every opportunity.

If you've sought to lovingly trust the Lord through a miscarriage or the loss of a newborn baby, do you still find yourself fearing you may doubt God when that "test" date comes? Do you fear giving in to anger or depression? I certainly did.

I wondered: *What could be done to keep Satan at bay—and rise above my own tendency to retreat into self-pity—on what had been our baby's due date? How could a day destined for sorrow— perhaps anger—be turned around? Was it okay to still experience grief, even if my hope and prayer was to experience spiritual victory on that day?*

Have any of those questions crossed *your* mind? Can we have a reasonable hope for success, or must we simply resign ourselves to doing our best to merely survive the day?

❧

Do you remember that sweet-sounding word we discussed in earlier chapters: *Victory?* Is it possible for an ordinary Christian to walk in victory on *that* day?

December 5th was our lost baby's due date, and as the day drew closer I found myself more and more in prayer about it. I didn't *want* to hand Satan a victory on that day! I longed to live in the power of Christ and be spiritually pure.

Months earlier, when the miscarriage occurred, I hoped I would be expecting another baby by the time our lost baby's due date arrived. That didn't happen. Not only was I not pregnant, the timing was wrong for me to even consider I *might* become pregnant during that particular week.

While praying, it occurred to me I was preparing for a strong defense against Satan's attacks on December 5th. But God caused me to recognize that, as opposed to digging down into a defensive position, I could be launched into an offensive strike. God was fully able to do more than just help me survive the day *if* I was willing to come before Him and set it apart as a special day; a day which was holy; a day in which I would pray for others.

I recognized there would be tears in the process, and felt this was not only okay but appropriate.

⁂

What? Satan tried to intervene. *Why should you pray for anyone else on your lost baby's due date? That will be a hard day for you! Pray for others? Don't be ridiculous! It's your day of grief!*

God was so faithful, so close to me as I prayed about setting apart December 5th as a holy day of prayer. I remember thinking about God and His love for me and other women who needed comfort. I knew there had to be women scattered throughout the world who had shared the same due date with me who also faced the despair of miscarriage. At that moment I committed to making our baby's due date a day set apart for prayer for others experiencing infertility.

❧

While I had a few responsibilities to deal with on that December day, I was able to set it apart for prayer. Multiple times I thought about and prayed for other women who had been or were going through that dark, dark valley of irreplaceable loss. My own experience of pain sharply brought to mind what others had experienced or perhaps were experiencing that very day.

God broadened my vision and compassion as I prayed. I needed no faces or names. I knew there were living, breathing women all over the world who felt alone in their pain that day; women who were crying tears, desiring a baby, and feeling despair. Tears flowed freely.

I asked for the Spirit of God to comfort those who, like me, lost a baby who was due on that date. I was moved to pray for those women who were miscarrying *that day*, for those who might be "fertile" *that day*, and for those who were disappointed by a menstrual cycle or negative pregnancy test *that day*. My plea and request was that God, in His wisdom and sovereignty, would work in a powerful way in the life of each of His dear children who suffered from infertility *that day*. I prayed God might heal a troubled pregnancy, encourage weak hearts, and open and close the doors of wombs as He saw fitting and best *that day*.

What could have been a day of spiritual shipwreck became one of close, intimate communion with God, a day in which

He graciously allowed me to minister to others. I found in so doing, God's love for *all* of us filled me with awe. It served to gift me with a fresh understanding of how incredibly merciful God really is. The quietest of miracles enfolded me.

I wondered if there would be a time in heaven the Lord Himself might joyfully bring each woman around I prayed for that day and say, "June! This is Jacqueline! You interceded on her behalf on December 5th. Now I will let *her* tell you how mightily I worked in her life that day." I may or may not ever know all the ways in which God honored my prayers on that special day, and it really doesn't matter. What I was *not* prepared for, however, was what happened to an acquaintance I had been ministering to in previous months.

Allie and her husband had started seeing an infertility specialist after some prodding and encouragement from me. They didn't see the specialist as an answer to prayer. They hated how clinical everything had become, and while I empathized with her and understood their frustration, I urged them to continue praying about it and just try using the specialist a little bit longer. I had spent countless hours on the phone with this dear Christian as she cried her heart out about her desire to have children. Then one day Allie told me they were quitting the medical route. While I found their decision to be a little disappointing, I *fully* understood. We hadn't visited with each other for a while, so I called her one afternoon to let her know I was thinking about her and to see how she was doing. "June, you will *never* believe what has happened!" Allie told me. As it turned out, she was expecting! I was beside myself with joy.

I learned Allie and Sean had decided to try one more time to see about conceiving with the help of the infertility specialist. She told me the doctor stated, "Well, we're cutting the timing of this awfully close. If you get pregnant, it will *definitely* be today. Probably within the next four hours." Do you know what she said next?

"June, I will never forget December 5th as long as I live!"

I was stunned. "Why?" I asked weakly.

"Because that's the day we had the procedure done!"

I was so blown away by the power of God, I laughed and cried at the same time. "Praise the Lord! Oh, praise God!" I exclaimed.

Two weeks later, Allie and Sean learned they were not expecting one baby, but *two!*

⁊⫶

It still thrills me whenever I think about it. How specific and clear was *that?!* God is so amazing. This apprehensive woman conceived on December 5th, with *twins.*

⁊⫶

It almost seemed as though God came down, intimately embraced me, and said, "Wasn't that affirming, June, My love? That second baby, by the way, is a living reminder of your child, who is with Me; your child who never knew a harsh word, never knew a moment's pain, and with whom you will spend eternity in My glorious kingdom!"

⁊⫶

What God did on that special day of prayer was far above anything I could have imagined. My friend, this heartbroken sister in Christ Jesus, became a joyful mother of a little boy and girl. What a *victory!* And I felt—well, actually knew—God graciously permitted me to be His special partner in that amazing miracle. The *first* miracle God performed—for the blessing of prayer and close fellowship with Him on a day Satan surely hoped would derail me—would have been more than enough for me. Yet God poured out one blessing on top of another in flagrant generosity.

❧

I'm convinced, dear friend, that most of us do *not* have a good handle on what God is willing to do through weak, ordinary people who are willing to pray on the behalf of others. But I know in my heart God did all kinds of miracles on that day of prayer. Why He let me in on one of them before reaching heaven I don't know, but it certainly has fueled my faith and convinced me that earnest, intercessory prayer is never wasted. I have a feeling some of heavens' treasures will include learning and seeing the mighty things God did *through* us while we were walking in this broken world.

❧

I hesitated to share this story because I know some of you might be discouraged because it seems as if your prayers are bouncing off the ceiling and God is steadfastly and conspicuously silent for reasons known only to Him. I personally know how painful it is when we see or hear of fantastic things God is doing in the lives of other people and wonder if, perhaps, something is wrong with us because we're in what seems like a long, painful spell of unanswered prayer.

This is when we must cling to God and His promises, trust Him by choice, and believe *He* is at work. We can boldly pray something along the lines of, "Lord God, I don't see how You are working, but I want to thank You for the fact that You *are*. And Your work is beautiful, and I know it will be revealed to the whole of creation in due time."

I have no doubt God will one day reveal to us His miraculous workings which were occurring during the "silent" times He led us through, and He will do so at the perfect time and in the perfect way.

Here is what I accept as true and believe that our heavenly Father wants us to know:

❋ He cares about you;

❋ He cares about your unborn child(ren);

❋ He cares about others you can relate to;

❋ He hears the cry of the broken hearted;

❋ The prayers of a righteous man or woman (normal, committed believer) can accomplish much (James 5:16);

❋ He is ready and willing to bless you; and

❋ Miracles will pour out as a direct result of your prayers even if you aren't able to identify a single one; even if your prayers seem to be met by a wall of silence from God. It's sometimes in our times of greatest darkness and heartache that God is doing the greatest work in our lives and in the lives of those we are praying for.

Our great and mighty God does *not* promise to show us all His workings and answers to prayer this side of heaven. However, I do believe if we commit to serve others and set aside our due dates as days of prayer, *we* will be blessed, even though receiving a blessing for ourselves is not our motivation.

When we pray with the mind of Christ, we are worshipping and remembering God: Remembering who He is and what He has done. Unselfishly praying for others and worshipping God will *never* leave us with a hurt or bitter heart, and therein lies our key for victory on that day, or any other day in the year the pangs hit us.

As we draw close to our Creator in prayer, *we* will be reminded of God's sovereignty and love. We will remember the hurts we feel are felt by others and that God has not forgotten *any* of us. We'll catch a better glimpse of the Father and be comforted to know He will one day raise us up in glory and joy. And He Himself will wipe our tears away.

> For I consider that the sufferings of this present time are not worthy to be compared with the glory that is to be revealed to us. (Romans 8:18)

When I consider the depth and intensity of some of our sufferings, I find myself confessing the glory to come is beyond my ability to grasp.

If you have lost any children, I weep because of your pain and am grieved by your grief. It is my prayerful petition the Father will touch you with healing.

❧

You may not feel ready to march into victory right now. Perhaps, today, your need is to be pulled from the front line of battle and be ministered to. Just trying to read through your tears may be the best you can do at this time. But will you let God's Word wash over you?

Consider Psalm 119:25-32, with my commentary in italics:

My soul cleaves to the dust.
> *This really hurts, God.*

Revive me according to Your word.
> *You and Your Word are the only absolutes I can rely on right now.*

I have told of my ways,
> *You're allowing me to grieve.*

And You have answered me.
> *You have acknowledged there is cause for my grief; You have answered me when I needed Your reassurance.*

Teach me Your statutes.
> *I still need to be taught about You, Lord.*

Make me understand the way of Your precepts,
> *I need and desire understanding. Help me understand the path and the nature of Your laws for me—what my standards should be.*

So I will meditate on Your wonders.
> *Then I'll find myself mulling over the indescribable works of Your hands. This will strengthen me and fill me with praise.*

My soul weeps because of grief;
> *This loss still hurts, God. Even when I'm done crying on the outside, I'm still weeping deep in my heart.*

Strengthen me according to Your word.

> *You love me even when I'm sick with grief.*
> *Because of that, I feel I can ask You to build me*
> *back up. You can equip me with everything I need*
> *through Your recorded Word. Employ Your Word*
> *and Spirit to restore me. Your Word will help me*
> *when nothing else can.*

Remove the false way from me,

> *The dark untruths I'm tempted to ponder are not*
> *what I need or want. Cause them to flee; make*
> *them foreign and unfamiliar to my heart.*

And graciously grant me Your law.

> *In place of those falsehoods, give me Your desires*
> *for my life. Your rules and admonishments are*
> *given because of Your mercy and grace; pour them*
> *out on me in love.*

I have chosen the faithful way;

> *I'm going to stick with you, God.*

I have placed Your ordinances before me.

> *Your goals for me have become my goals for myself.*
> *With great deliberateness, I'm focusing on You and*
> *Your game plan alone.*

I cleave to Your testimonies;

> *Like a drowning man, I'm clinging to Your*
> *recorded promises as if they were a life-raft.*

O Lord, do not put me to shame!

> *I'm putting all my eggs in Your basket, God.*
> *The world is watching. Show them that it pays to*
> *trust in You!*

I shall run in the way of Your commandments,

> *I've decided that I'm not going to go after this half-heartedly, God. I'm going to run, strain, and exert myself to follow after You.*

For You will enlarge my heart.

> *Because You, O great God, will strengthen and enable me to do this. You will make me wiser and stronger. My heart will expand to accommodate the added treasures You will pour upon me.*

ॐ

MY PRAYER FOR YOU: Father God, this beloved child may know you as Lord, as Savior, as Friend, as Defender, and I praise and thank You for that. I pray she will intimately know you as her Healer, and that You will be the lifter of her head and the encourager of her heart.

17

Secondary Infertility: Disgustingly New or Déjà Vu

WHETHER A COUPLE ACHIEVED a successful pregnancy after much work, expense, and trouble or conceived and carried their first child with relative ease, they share the heartbreak of secondary infertility when it becomes obvious a younger sibling for their son or daughter isn't happening. Secondary infertility is the inability to conceive or safely carry a baby to full term after having succeeded in having one or more children biologically.

If you're one of those couples who had problems the first time around, one of your worst fears is realized: "We're having this nightmare *again?*"

If you're a couple who finds it to be a new problem, I'm sure you experienced some genuine bewilderment: "Us? You've got to be *kidding!*"

A friend of mine had no problem whatsoever with conception and the safe delivery of their first two children. They were one of those enviable couples who could plan a romantic evening and have their desired baby approximately nine months later. This friend was sympathetic toward the women she knew who were in the furnace of infertility, even though she had never experienced it. When Baby Number Three failed to materialize for her and her husband, it was a bit of a surprise. When long months passed and Baby Number Three *still* didn't show up for the party, it had become shockingly painful.

If you've battled infertility initially and are now experiencing it again, you likely have some repeat struggles to deal with in addition to several new ones. For example, many couples who underwent infertility and finally, successfully birthed a baby believed their delight and gratitude to God for one child would always be sufficient for them. Maybe this was your experience, but as your baby grows and somehow becomes even more precious and enjoyable, it may not be long before there is an intense desire to have another baby; not only for your own enjoyment but to provide one or more siblings for your *child* to benefit from and grow up with.

Perhaps you've assumed you wouldn't be wrestling with the old *Why me?* question again after having suffered infertility and then experienced the miracle and blessings of having a child.

"If God never gives us another baby," a friend of mine who had experienced infertility testified, "we won't complain! We are just so fortunate to have our daughter. She is precious! We are blessed beyond our dreams." Not even two years later, however, this same friend was "too hurt and angry" to pray to her heavenly Father. Why? Because she and her husband were unable to fulfill their natural desire for another child. They had *assumed* their painful infertility days were behind them or, that because of the thrill from past victories, their trust in God would never again falter. Nonetheless, all the loneliness, fear, anger, rebellion, and pain this friend had encountered *before* was now back in full force. It caught both her and her husband off-guard.

If you've made an incorrect assumption that your contentment with one child would shield you from further infertility pain or anger, you may have to work through those trust lessons you already wrestled through with God.

This reminds me of board games when you land on the wrong square and have to go back to start. Even as an adult, I find it annoying to play a game and get stuck going back to where I've already been. It's frustrating, *especially* with infertility; and it can carry a ferocious price in time and emotions.

What if you find yourself right back where you started from, only to realize you played the "infertility game" poorly the first time around (no matter how your first child came to you)? I humbly offer that if you manage to skip "buying into" the important foundations we addressed in earlier chapters through infertility, you will not be in good shape to withstand the furnace blast of secondary infertility. *Now* is the time to stop, reevaluate where you are, and start again with a learner's heart. Why? Because you'll be incomparably better off if you can bring yourself to embrace the following:

* *God's answer to "Why?"*
* *A restored relationship with Him*
* *Victory through stubborn obedience*
* *A worthy life goal*
* *A solid support structure*
* *Unwavering reliance on God and His Word*

You cannot take any shortcuts through life's trials and expect to grow and be strengthened in your spirit. There are no true shortcuts to true refinement. If we try, we unfortunately open the door to more suffering.

Secondary infertility provides a grueling testing ground for strengthening one's Christian walk. How you or I handle infertility the second time around depends on how well we understood and embraced what God was working to teach us the *first* time around.

Do you need to go back to start? One good thing about it if you do: God is right there waiting in perfect love to help you.

❧

As touched on earlier, people who haven't experienced infertility are sometimes insensitive to those struggling with it. Yet those of us who *do* struggle with infertility can be somewhat insensitive to those who are secondary infertility strugglers.

Oh, no! You may think. *Here she goes meddling with our heart issues again, when we're the walking wounded!* Honestly, I get that. But haven't you found your thoughts running along lines such as these? "At least they have one child to enjoy! We haven't even got that." Or, "They don't have it so rough. I'd be happy to be in their shoes." Those have been my thoughts on more than one occasion.

If we assess *ourselves* honestly, we may find we who have no children can occasionally be insensitive to those who are experiencing secondary infertility. Of course, this is an uncomfortable thought. We want others to be sensitive and understanding toward *us!* Of all people, however, we should be the most compassionate and understanding of another woman or couple longing for another baby. Perhaps like me you need to occasionally evaluate your compassion level and prayer support toward anyone you know who desires another child and is not seeing that hope realized. These same shoes may one day be on our own feet. Couples experiencing secondary infertility need our love and support far more than we realize.

⁂

Thank you for permitting me to take that important detour before addressing another assumption common with couples who suffered through infertility prior to having a child: *A baby happened for us before; it will happen for us again.*

Many times this is true. For some women, getting pregnant and having a child seems to help "clear up" whatever problem they had encountered with infertility, and they go on from there falling into the more "normal" ranges of conception and healthy pregnancies. I wish this would be the case for everyone; however, it isn't.

If things haven't cleared up, another pregnancy has not occurred, or if you've never had an infertility problem until now, you're likely considering your options while delighting in the child you already gave birth to. You observe and study your child thoughtfully. You despair. It may be difficult to imagine adopting your next one. Should you seriously consider it? Things surely wouldn't turn out so well, would they? Ah, do I see another possible assumption rearing its head?

Actually, adoption can be an *easier* consideration after having one biological child. Some couples find being parents even more enjoyable than they had anticipated, their biological child to be more unique and individual from themselves than they would have believed, and they don't care to waste precious years and resources in what could be a futile pursuit of pregnancy.

They're thinking this kid stuff is pretty fantastic, and it doesn't matter how they come.

If a couple is *more* uncomfortable with thoughts of adoption after having their first child biologically, this is also understandable. It's possible to assume the biological child will be healthier or, blush to think, more intelligent than one they didn't conceive or carry. Thinking people may wonder if it would be fair to raise an adopted child alongside their biological child in case they are dissimilar to one another. Whether or not considered valid, these kinds of concerns add to the stress of secondary infertility. Don't beat up on yourself if you're having such fears; but please… know that such concerns are based on *assumptions*.

Why do I address assumptions we can make regarding secondary infertility as if they are undesirable? Simply this: assumptions have the power to usher in some of the greatest mistakes we make in our lives; mistakes which generate sorrow in the long run. For this reason, I'm hoping you'll permit me to ask your consideration of the following question: If you are basing important family decisions on assumptions, will you prayerfully take them to the Lord?

Among the many other struggles relating to infertility, secondary infertility has an added heartache: a child—your child—may share in your longing for another baby.

A mother experiencing secondary infertility told me of the recent time she had a friend over for a visit. Her five-year-old was fascinated with their guest's body as she was eight months' pregnant.

"I explained to my daughter that our friend had a baby growing in her tummy, and she became very excited. Her daughter's next words were, 'Is there a baby in *your* tummy too, Mommy?'"

Even retelling the story was difficult for this wonderful, Christian mother. "No," she explained with patience and pain. "There isn't, honey."

"But you would *like* to have a baby in your tummy, wouldn't you?"

By this time both women were fighting tears.

"Yes, I would," came her admission from the heart. Her daughter then suggested they pray about it, on the spot. So the three of them did. After praying, amidst the silent tears of her mother and friend, the little girl looked up with bright expectation as she gently touched her mother's abdomen.

"Is there a baby in your tummy *now*, Mommy?"

To me, that would most definitely fit in a "highly difficult to deal with" category.

Friends and family members may be assuming you'll be pregnant again before long or may think you're an ingrate for not being content with the child you have; perhaps they're opposed to your desire to pursue adoption. And all this may be taking place while you, perhaps, are doing your best to answer some *very* tough questions from your son or daughter.

A hundred hurts, in a hundred different ways.

"Can you tell me again why we can't have a baby? I forgot."

"Is there a baby in your tummy now, Mommy?"

❧

Whether it is disgustingly new or dèjá vu, secondary infertility *is* rife with pain.

If this is where you find yourself at this time, please know there is no shame in acknowledging the pain and continuing to petition God in prayer for additional children. Also, in deep love, please permit me to encourage you to be wise and courageous in dealing with the dangers of assumptions.

It's my hope you will pray, plan, and commit to enlarging your family. While doing so, thoughtfully assess the condition of your support structure, that important life goal which isn't dependent upon circumstances, and the application of God's Word in the face of reality that we covered in earlier chapters. Possessing a strong grip on the truths we have already shared together will enable you to better enjoy and parent the child you've been entrusted with as you eagerly await the Master's perfect plan to unfold before you regarding your family.

My friend, pray for victory one skirmish at a time and for the ability to remember God's truths, which will help you. Hug your little one, consistently whispering and teaching amazing truths of God into his or her little ears.

Perhaps you noticed back in chapter 13, where I quoted Psalm 113, that God addresses barren women: "He makes the barren woman abide in the house as a joyful mother of children. Praise the Lord!" (Psalm 113:9). Note the use of the plural: *children.*

Together, let's praise the Lord that He has that kind of power. And while thanking Him for it, do *not* be afraid to ask Him to permit this Bible verse to describe *you* if it will bring added honor and glory to Him.

❧

Praise the LORD. How good it is to sing praises to our God, how pleasant and fitting to praise Him! The LORD builds up Jerusalem; He gathers the exiles of Israel. He heals the brokenhearted, and binds up their wounds. He determines the number of the stars and calls them each by name. Great is our LORD and mighty in power; His understanding has no limit. The LORD sustains the humble but casts the wicked to the ground. Sing to the LORD with grateful praise; make music to our God on the harp. He covers the sky with clouds; He supplies the earth with rain and makes grass grow on the hills. He provides food for the cattle, and for the young ravens when they call. His pleasure is not in the strength of the horse, nor His delight in the legs of the warrior; the LORD delights in those who fear him, who put their hope in His unfailing love. (Psalm 147:1-11, NIV)

Did you know you were on God's mind when He had Scripture penned, dear one? Let Him pour His words of love and encouragement over you as you enjoy your child and seek His face for another.

A number of the Bible's outstanding people of faith were ordinary men and women who knew heartache, repeatedly sought to honor God, and openly petitioned Him for a child. God often sets a dramatic stage before He publicly displays a great and miraculous work.

⁂

MY PRAYER FOR YOU: You've reminded me today, Lord, that prayer is not just a method for us to tell You what it is we hope You'll do. It's another tool for intimacy with You in which our hearts are often changed and we are stilled to hear Your Word and Your voice. If this reader is suffering through secondary infertility, I know You care about every detail of her and her little family's life. I pray You will give her a song and a heart of wisdom, even in her pain. I ask for her faith and trust to be multiplied—and that she will have confidence You are setting the stage for a beautiful, powerful work in her and her family's life. Thank You.

18

How Do You Pray?

PRAYER! It's such an important aspect of the believer's life, yet often misunderstood.

We were signed up for adoption and in the waiting stage before beginning the agency's classes on certification. We had been on the waiting list for several months and figured we would be eligible for placement of a baby sometime during the next calendar year. Additionally, we had been seeing the infertility specialist for several months, going through the infertility "workout."

Through this season, we shared our prayer requests with other believers in Jesus Christ.

Pinpointing our infertility problem didn't come easily; only a cervical mucus problem cropped up from time to time. Our specialist had received a great deal of publicity for contributing to advances in the field, and we hoped we could take full advantage of his expertise.

Our wish eventually came true. The doctor suggested we try an advanced insemination surgery, called a lower tubal transfer;

we were pleased. We shared with others who had been praying for us what we were going to be doing, and *that* is when the confusion and chaos about prayer began.

It was incredible!

I had already "built my altar" (as shared earlier) and expressed my trust to God. Not trust that He would give us children, just *trust*—whether He chose to give us children or not. Even though we longed to have a baby and were zealously pursuing our options for becoming parents, I was experiencing amazing peace of mind.

We began preparing for the procedure. I had to take fertility drugs orally and by shots. As a couple, we prayed every day that God's will would be done.

One by one, people began to tell me—nicely, of course—that I was praying too cautiously. They maintained I had to pray with unwavering faith that God would honor the surgery and cause me to become pregnant. They were quite adamant that praying for God's will to be done was a sign of weak faith. This was a bit shocking to hear; my experience was *completely* the opposite.

It took far greater faith for me to pray for God's will to be done than *mine!*

Yet another small group of people took me aside and told me they *already knew* I was going to get pregnant from the procedure. I asked them how they knew in advance what God was going to do? They told me it was because I *deserved* it. I found myself gently asking: "So, what you're saying is God *owes* me a pregnancy?"

I vividly recall one woman's puzzled expression when I asked this question. She responded, "Well, it doesn't sound good the way *you* say it, but God is going to let you get pregnant from the surgery because you're such a nice Christian girl and God wouldn't allow you to suffer any more than you already have. Besides," she reasoned with a furrowed brow, "we're *all* praying for it to work!"

"Do you mean God has absolutely *no choice* but to give us a pregnancy in the next four weeks?" I asked.

Here this poor saint was trying to encourage me, and she probably felt as though I was bent on provoking her. Actually, I *did* want to do some provoking: of her thinking about the person of God.

I began praying my Christian friends and acquaintances with this narrow view of God would have *their* faith stretched and see that God is limitless in His ways.

My concern about people and prayer reached new heights two days later when *another* Christian friend told me I was going to get pregnant from our procedure. "Why is that?" I asked bluntly. She responded with closed fists and tight face, "Because, God has to make it work, June. He just *has* to!"

I hope you can understand my growing dilemma. I *was* hoping God would give us a baby. But I also longed for God to show these caring people He did *not* have to prove He was God by jumping through a hoop like some kind of trained seal.

If we want to avoid errors or shallowness in praying to God, we need to know the answers to some critically important questions, which typically don't flash across our radars.

QUESTION 1:
WHAT KIND OF FAITH PLEASES GOD?

One cannot read the Bible without finding the importance of having faith or belief. Consider these verses: Matthew 21:22, Romans 14:23, Hebrews 11:6, Romans 4:19-20, and Hebrews 11:1-2. *Faith pleases God!*

Perhaps you, like me, often mistake feelings for faith. Because I was not 100 percent certain God would use the surgical procedure to give us a child, a few people who cared for me believed this to mean I was lacking in faith. These friends felt I needed to ask specifically for a surgery which resulted in pregnancy (that is, to name what I wanted of God) and then have complete faith God would do as I asked (that is, to claim He would come through with it). When faith is applied in this manner, however, it can create a dangerous breeding ground for placing one's faith in faith instead of placing one's *faith* in *God*.

God does *not* want us to have faith in our faith. He wants us to have faith in Him.

The kind of faith which pleases God is that which may say, "My Lord and God, I don't understand, but I accept whatever it is You want to do in and through me. And I praise You for Your good and perfect ways."

QUESTION 2:
WHAT ARE GOD'S ATTRIBUTES (CHARACTERISTICS)?

Of all the pages of this book perhaps the next few are the ones the enemy of God and His people wants us to skip, rush through, or misunderstand the most. If we gain even the slightest understanding of each of God's attributes, we'll possess such awe, confidence in, and love for Him that Satan's lies and schemes against us will become utterly useless. For this reason, we are entering into a holy battleground. Will you please stop in your reading right now and ask God to help you understand better who and what He is? Thank you so much.

God Is Spirit. The Bible puts this into clear focus for us: "God is Spirit, and His worshippers must worship in spirit and in truth" (John 4:24). The word *spirit* used here derives from the Greek word *pneuma*, which means a current of air that is a breath or a breeze. It connotes *rationalization* and mental disposition—in other words, clear, rational thinking. *Pneuma* comes from the root word *pneo*, which means "to breathe hard" or "to blow, a *forcible respiration*." God is a life-giving breath which provides not only life itself but balance and rational thought. We are therefore able to respond to Him in worship with our lives with clear, rational minds. When I first came to grasp what it really means that *God is spirit*, I blurted out loud: "*Wow!*"

God Is Unity. The shema states, "Hear O Israel! The Lord is our God, the Lord is one" (Deuteronomy 6:4). Jesus said to the Jews in the temple, "I and the Father are one" (John 10:30). The resurrected Christ commanded His followers to make disciples of all the nations, "baptizing them in the name [singular] of the Father, and the Son and the Holy Spirit" (Matthew 28:19). What does God's unity provide to us? God's unity validates the ministry of Christ and the Holy Spirit. If Christ were not God, there would be no avenue of salvation for the sinful human. If the Holy Spirit were not God, we would have no breath of life or rational thought. There would be no Heavenly Father, no God the Son, and no Comforter. There wouldn't be an avenue for us to access God's love, or for His love to reach us. As you can see, any watered down version of God the Father, God the Son, and God the Holy Spirit in perfect unity (oneness) is horrific. How we should thank and adore God for His unity!

God Is Infinite. He is without termination or end. God declares, "I am the Alpha and the Omega, who is, and who was, and who is to come, the Almighty" (Revelation 1:8). The word *alpha* is the first letter of the Greek alphabet and means "first." *Omega* is the last letter, and means "end." The psalmist declares:

> Of old You founded the earth, and the heavens are the work of Your hands. Even they will perish, but You endure; and all of them will wear out like a garment; like clothing You will change them and they will be changed. But You are the same, and Your years will not come to an end. (Psalm 102:25-27)

We will never lose our God and King! He is infinite! We see things wearing out (or people bailing out) everywhere around us. What a comfort to know the God we approach in prayer is not "here today and gone tomorrow." No faithlessness on our part can dislodge Him. No question or pronouncements of people can cause Him to cease to exist.

God Is Eternal. He is free from the restrictions of time. You and I are time watchers. Our biological clocks keep ticking, we want a baby, and we wonder if God has lost track of time. Yet Psalm 90:1-2 shows the Lord has been our dwelling place in all generations and goes on to say, "before the mountains were born or You gave birth to the earth and the world, even from everlasting to everlasting, You are God." Time, therefore, is not our enemy but God's tool. God and His purposes are not bound or restricted by time—even if we think they are!

God Is Immutable. He is unchanging and unchangeable. James tells us "Every good thing given and every perfect gift is from above, coming down from the Father of lights, with whom there is no variation, or shifting shadow" (James 1:17). What we call our circumstances (what we see) does not change the perfection and truth of God. He is unchanging. How horrible it would be if God were like us: reliable one day and failing the next, or kind-intentioned toward us most of the time but stabbing us in the back at others. What a solid foundation we have in our God who is everything He says He is in His Word—all the time!

God Is Omnipresent. This means He is everywhere. We cannot successfully run or hide from Him, neither can we be blocked *from* Him by any person, power, or circumstance. What a comfort and a thrill this truth should be for us! The psalmist lays it out clearly:

> Where can I go from Your Spirit? Or where can I flee
> from Your presence? If I ascend to heaven, You are there;
> if I make my bed in Sheol, behold, You are there. If I
> take the wings of the dawn, if I dwell in the remotest
> part of the sea, even there Your hand will lead me, and
> Your right hand will lay hold of me. (Psalm 139:7-10)

God is personally present with the sinner on his knees asking Him for forgiveness at the same time He is present with His child suffering persecution thousands of miles away. He is with *you*. We don't have to be in a special building or have a certain person intercede for us in order to have immediate and constant fellowship and interaction with God. Mind-boggling, isn't it?

God Is Sovereign. In other words, He is the Supreme Ruler. God is in control even when things may appear otherwise. Psalm 66:7 is one example of many Scriptures where God's sovereignty is highlighted: "He rules by His might forever; His eyes keep watch on the nations; Let not the rebellious exalt themselves." God does not have to maneuver. He doesn't have to counter maneuver. He never has to go to a Plan B. He has no slips of control. He is orchestrating the events of mankind, including every detail of your life and mine. This makes the posturing of arrogant people a parade of foolishness while serving to remove fear from the hearts of His beloved children—even in the midst of life's fiercest storms.

God Is Omniscient. In other words, God knows all actual and possible things. He not only knows everything going on, everything which has occurred in the past, and everything which will happen in the future, but everything which *would* have happened if certain things *had happened!* In the cities and communities in which Christ performed many of His miracles (yet where the people did not repent), He said to them, "Woe to you, Chorazin! Woe to you, Bethsadia! For if the miracles had occurred in Tyre and Sidon which occurred in you, they would have repented long ago in sackcloth and ashes" (Matthew 11:21). What a blessing to have an all-powerful, all-loving God we can approach in prayer who is not lacking any necessary, firsthand knowledge!

God Is Omnipotent. He is all powerful. God cannot be hindered, intimidated, or blackmailed. There is nothing He chooses to do for which He does not have the power to implement. Wow! What if He were all powerful and *not* holy? Or what if He were all powerful and *not* unchanging? God will take care of all business which needs to be taken care of.

Wrongs which have occurred on the earth will one day be made right. "Then I heard something like the voice of a great multitude and like the sound of many waters and like the sound of mighty peals of thunder, saying, 'Hallelujah! For the Lord our God, the Almighty, reigns.'" (Revelation 19:6).

God Is Just. "He has fixed a day in which He will judge the world in righteousness through a Man whom He has appointed, having furnished proof to all men by raising Him from the dead" (Acts 17:31). God will personally judge and enact *vengeance* where it is due. Romans 12:19 gives me chills: "Never take your own revenge, beloved, but leave room for the wrath of God, for it is written, 'Vengeance is Mine, I will repay,' says the Lord." God's justice also includes *forgiveness!* "If we confess our sins, He is faithful and *just* to forgive us our sins and to cleanse us from all unrighteousness" (1 John 1:9). We should take huge measures of healthy fear *and* comfort in the truth that God is just!

God Is Love. He is love through and through; it's not something He has to apply, practice, or work Himself up to. His incomprehensible plan of salvation is the supreme example:

> But God, being rich in mercy, for His great love with which He loved us, even when we were dead in our transgressions, made us alive together with Christ (by grace you have been saved) and raised us up with Him, and seated us with Him in the heavenly places in Christ Jesus. (Ephesians 2:4-6)

Simply put: *We would all be toast were it not for God's intentional, active love and His "impossible to understand" mercy.* John 3:16 never grows old: "For God so loved the world, that He gave His only begotten Son, that whoever believes in Him shall not perish, but have eternal life." God *is* love whether or not people choose to believe in Him or respond to His love.

God Is Truth. God is true in all that He does; He is consistent with Himself. Jesus said, "I am the way, and the truth, and the life: no one comes to the Father but through Me" (John 14:6). God and God alone is the source of truth. "You, O Lord, will not withhold Your compassion from me; Your loving-kindness and Your truth will continually preserve me" (Psalm 40:11). Rock solid encouragement and breathtaking hope is rooted in truth—the trustworthiness—of God. And He has not been stingy in revealing truth to us. We can read truth about God and from God in the Bible from cover to cover. We can lean on it daily. We can rely on it and claim it in our every battle.

God Is Free. This attribute means God is independent from His creatures. "Who has directed the Spirit of the Lord, or as His counselor has informed Him? With whom did He consult and who gave Him understanding? And who taught Him in the path of justice and taught Him knowledge and informed Him in the way of understanding?" (Isaiah 40:13-14). This is another beautiful attribute of God's! He loves us; He is Truth. He is in control, and He does not need us to tell Him how to function. He doesn't need our advice. He is not dependent upon our input or opinion to be who He is. How incredibly *refreshing!*

God Is Holy. The Hebrew word for holy means "apartness, set-apartness." God is separate and apart from all else—above all else. This is the only one of God's attributes the Bible places together *three* times:

> In the year of King Uzziah's death, I saw the LORD sitting on a throne, lofty and exalted, with the train of

His robe filling the temple. Seraphim stood above Him, each having six wings; with two he covered his face, and with two he covered his feet, and with two he flew. And one called out to another and said, "Holy, Holy, Holy is the LORD of hosts. The whole earth is full of his glory." And the foundations of the thresholds trembled at the voice of him who called out, while the temple was filling with smoke. (Isaiah 6:1-4)

God's holiness is to be both appreciated by His dear children and feared by all. It's His all-consuming holiness which demanded a *perfect* sacrifice for the sins of the world. The flippant, the braggarts, and those who are practicing religion and relying on good works to win approval from God will be in absolute terror before Him and His all-consuming holiness.

I'm not a Bible scholar, but I believe there's another awe-inspiring attribute of God's that needs to be trumpeted.

God Is Personal. God desires to have relationship with His creation. The Triune God desired to create man in His own image with the ability to fellowship (see Genesis 1:26). He personally formed man out of the dust and then amazingly put His *mouth* on a face made of *dirt* and breathed life into him (see Genesis 2:7). From the first book of the Bible through the last, God invites anyone who wants to have peace, eternal life, and intimacy with God to come to Him. God is with those who become His children through faith in Jesus Christ and promises to never leave them or forsake them. He is preparing a home for those who love Him and walk with Him on this earth to be *with Him* in glory (see John 14:1-3). He knows us by name (see Revelation 3:5). He knows the number of hairs on our head, an ever-changing sum (see Matthew 10:30). He calls us His children (see Romans 8:16). He calls us His heirs (see Romans 8:17). He calls us His friends (see John 15:15). God is personal towards those who oppose Him as well. We saw earlier that vengeance belongs to God. He will personally judge those who reject His provision for the forgiveness of sins and for salvation (see Revelation 20:11-13). If someone is an enemy to God's children, they have made themselves an enemy of God Himself. He is personal indeed!

In light of God's attributes, how can we do anything other than humble ourselves in worship and confess that God alone is holy and worthy of all our praise and all of our trust every day and every hour? This is the One we are praying to, my friend!

It's no wonder that nowhere in the Bible are we commanded to *understand* God! However, we *are* regularly instructed throughout His Word to *trust* Him.

QUESTION 3:
WHAT DOES IT MEAN TO PRAY IN JESUS' NAME?

And whatever you ask in My name, that will I do, so that the Father may be glorified in the Son. If you ask Me anything in My name, I will do it. (John 14:13-14)

In that day you will not question Me about anything. Truly, truly, I say to you, if you ask the Father for anything in My name, He will give it to you. Until now you have asked for nothing in My name; ask, and you will receive, that your joy may be made full. (John 16:23-24).

Most of us think praying in Jesus' name is to add the words *In Jesus' name, amen* at the end of each prayer. It's a phrase we rarely contemplate or dwell on. But let's back up for just a moment and cover what may seem to be the obvious. Who is Jesus to you? Lord and master whom you live to serve? Or maybe friend or buddy who you want as your "blessing heavy-weight" in life?

I think most of us—if we're honest—prefer to have Jesus as a friend and buddy more than we do as lord and master. Have you ever been guilty of praying "in Jesus' name" in hopes of getting what you really want for your own pleasure rather than for a hunger to have the Father glorified in the Son, as Jesus laid out for us in John 14:13? Yeah, I sort of thought so. Same here!

I'll never forget one pastor's account of a fervor of praying in Jesus' name he and his wife observed. A certain young lady started attending their church, which was mainly comprised of college students. She was apparently a girl of astonishing, natural beauty. He said even if a person were not the type to notice a person's looks too much, they would notice her. Not surprisingly, several of the single college guys in the congregation appeared to be mysteriously stricken with a very pure, noble love for this young lady and began hot pursuit for her hand in marriage. Being good Christian lads, they even prayed about it! Their prayers were basically the same, according to the pastor:

> *"Dear God, please make her mine.*
> *I love her. Oh, please, God, please!*
> *I ask this in Jesus' name, amen."*

If these college boys were all *truly* praying in Jesus' name the way He was talking about in John chapters 14 and 16, they each would have received a *Yes* from God, and this poor gal would have been stuck with about eight husbands. Eight husbands, I might add, who had great eyesight but not the best spiritual understanding or depth.

It's quite obvious these lads were hoping for their buddy Jesus to give them the edge over the other fellows who were, of course, hoping the same thing for themselves. Each one of them was trying to twist God's will to match their own personal will, so he would get to have that beautiful babe for a wife.

The Bible clearly states there will be people appearing before God in the judgment who will claim to have prayed and performed miracles in the name of Jesus but whose hearts were far from God's heart. The vast distance between their hearts and His will be exposed when Jesus Himself declares He never knew them (see Matthew 7:21-23). So Christians *and* non-Christians may not be praying in Jesus' name even if they *think* they are.

Praying in Jesus' name, the way it's meant in the above verses, is a heart cry or affirmation of a believer's desire to see God the Father glorified through Jesus; they want to pray God's way instead of their own. *In Jesus' name* is meant to reflect our faithful stewardship and service to Jesus Christ, whose name we are representing and whose desires we are anxious to carry out.

QUESTION 4:
AM I PRAYING BIBLICALLY?

Speaking for myself, I confess I often pray in the character of June Strickler rather than in the character of God the Son. Christ was perfect (unselfish), making it difficult for me to effectively pattern myself and my prayer life after Him. He had eternal perspective; I most often have a temporal perspective. It seems His every prayer was for the benefit of others; mine are primarily for myself and a select group of people I care for because of *their* love for *me*. Christ's purpose for His every prayer and action, contrarily, was aimed at one thing: that His *Father* would receive glory.

In times when my prayers *do* harmonize with the character of Christ, it's always clear God is honoring those prayers and petitions. This is when I see answers to prayer which can best be described as wild and crazy, followed by mind-boggling wonder and joyous praise.

How about you? Are you praying biblically?

If you want to have a sweetly intimate, successful prayer life with God, study through the Gospels—Matthew, Mark, Luke, and John—and write down notes on the prayers of Christ. Compare the way you pray and the way the Lord Jesus prayed. If your driving desire is to have God the Father glorified, your prayers will reflect that. When such is the case, you are praying in the character of Jesus Christ, praying in His name. It's only during those times we are truly praying biblically.

Every prayer and request we offer up in the character of Jesus—that is, in His name—*will* be honored by God the Father. This provides the trusting believer with thrilling comfort when receiving a "No" or "Wait" answer from God— because He is giving a "Yes" answer to our greater prayer to do what most honors Him. This, my friend, showers us with peace when we wouldn't normally find it. It beats back the flames in the furnace heat of trials and testing, gifting us with breathtaking hope... even when things look as if they aren't going right *at all*.

Thy kingdom come;
Thy will be done;
On earth (including in my heart), just as it is in heaven.

MY PRAYER FOR YOU: Wow, God! What a reminder this chapter has been of Your perfection and how foolish it is of us to ever doubt Your goodness or power. In Jesus' wonderful name, I ask that my suffering friend will know You and trust You and that her eyes will be opened—either for the first time or anew—to the fact that prayer and communion with You is a holy, amazing adventure and privilege.

19

The Holy Hallelujah!

WE ESTABLISHED EARLIER that the Path of Victory is a sweaty hike for any child of God who chooses to walk it, whether or not struggling with undesired childlessness. We also looked at there being a direct correlation between our obedience to God and our ability to experience spiritual victory in tough situations. Nonetheless, an amazing fact many Christians are largely unaware of remains. We often make our daily struggle to live and walk in holiness and victory more difficult than it has to be. This, my friend, is where the *Holy Hallelujah* comes rolling out!

In chapter 4 I told you about what I called BIG Truths in a Little Box. They address God's provision for us from the *penalty of sin* (the past), the *power of sin* (the present), and the very *presence of sin* (the future). These truths can transform our lives when accepted and acted upon by faith.

As a child I accepted, by faith, God's gift of salvation through Christ's sacrificial death on the cross (the first truth), which released me from the *penalty* of my sin. At the same time, I joyfully accepted God's gift permitting me to spend eternity in heaven with Christ, free from the *presence* of sin (the third truth). I nonetheless failed to understand—and subsequently take hold of by faith—the second truth made possible by the work Christ completed on the cross of Calvary as shared in Romans 6. This was when Christ won the victory over the *power* of sin in us by crucifying our "old self" (or sin nature we inherited from Adam, see I Corinthians 15:22) to the cross *with Him* (see Romans 6:1-8).

I occasionally wondered: If my old self was crucified with Christ as the Apostle Paul taught, why then did I still struggle with sin? And why did Paul share he struggled with it too?

How does this "old self being crucified with Christ" thing really work?

Well, it starts with this basic: People did *not* survive Roman crucifixions, a cruel method of capital punishment. And neither did our old self. The Bible tells us it was crucified with Christ. Jesus rose from the grave in victory over death, praise His name! Yet the believer's crucified, old self did *not* (Romans 6:6-7). This is a wonderful truth to embrace, my friend.

With His precious blood, Jesus sacrificially paid the ransom to permanently release believers from the chains of their sin DNA. He won the victory once and for all over the horrific, gripping power of sin: the power we were *slaves* to. When sin whistled its summons, we were the slaves conditioned to answer.

Through a person's faith in the risen Jesus, this immediately changes. Yes, the Christ follower will have struggles with sin until his or her physical death and being welcomed into the presence of God (Romans 7:15). But he or she was released from the kingdom of darkness and its chains to sin through

Jesus and made an heir of God's kingdom of light and spiritual freedom.

When sin whistles now, the child of God has the freedom to *ignore its call*. The sin DNA that linked us to sin's taskmaster has been severed. Simply put, we are no longer its slaves (Romans 6:14). We belong in God's family and He bestowed on us the perfect, sinless DNA of Jesus.

This is *huge!* Through faith in Jesus, the *Sinner* label is no longer ours to wear. Jesus peeled it off and it's gone. A thing of the past.

Hallelujah!

❧

So how does this play out for the Christian? It means that if you and I are going to wallow in sin, we have to make a foolhardy attempt to remove that crucified, dead, old self off the cross, lay it out on the ground, and try to blow air into its decayed body. While this is a highly graphic and disturbing example, based on Romans chapter 6 any child of God choosing to sin is, in effect, trying to resuscitate a corpse.

❧

When I came to understand the significance of Christ having crucified our old self to His cross (Galatians 2:20), I was wild with joy and asked God to help me communicate how this truth practically *throws* us into victory over sin and temptation. Here's how He chose to answer that prayer:

> A stunning upset took place back in the 2000 Summer Olympics held in Sydney, Australia. A swimmer from

Equatorial Guinea came to represent his country, having learned to swim only eight short months prior to competing in the event. He had trained in a pool only 20 meters long and hadn't even seen a 50-meter Olympic pool until arriving in Sydney. This young man's times were painfully slow compared to his highly trained, skilled competitors. Some who watched him swimming feared he might even drown. Yet by the time his body pierced the water in what would become his winning swim, he knew beyond a shadow of a doubt he would be the Gold Medal winner of the Men's 100 Meter Freestyle event. And so did the crowd who watched it all unfold.

How did this happen? Strangely enough, victory was in reach before this unlikely champion's race even began because his rivals had made false starts. They were subsequently disqualified. A new race was set, so when the soon-to-be medalist made his winning swim he was the only athlete in the pool. He was the victor by default. (And he set a new Olympic record for the Men's 100 Meter Freestyle event—not for the fastest time, but the slowest.)

Although this man unexpectedly found himself free of competitors, he still had to exercise self-discipline, focus, and committed action to bring the victory to pass. In other words, he didn't jump into the Olympic Pool when it was time for the event to take place, splash around, and invite members of the crowd to come in and play water volleyball with him. Had he done so, he wouldn't have experienced the victory he did, nor would he have brought honor to his country.

This historical event (documented at The Olympic Museum in Lausanne, Switzerland) beautifully illustrates the truth about spiritual victory which most of us, as Christians, have lived far too long in ignorance of. We've sought for victory in given situations while failing to grasp the fact that—because of what Christ Jesus has completed on the cross—our victory is assured; in truth, it has *already occurred* (I Corinthians 15:57-58). We have been set free from the the chain of sin DNA.

Just as our Olympic swimmer was required to exercise self-discipline, focus, and action to *experience* victory, we must also. We must move forward—or stand firm—on the absolute conviction that what the Bible says Christ has accomplished on our behalf *has* been accomplished. And then we need to live like it. We commune with God's Holy Spirit and seek to walk in His ways. Our heart's desire is to live like sons and daughters of the Most High.

Through God's grace, we can swim in the painful events of infertility and fierce temptations, with all of their challenges. And even though our lungs may hurt, our noses and throats may burn with water, and we wonder whether we might actually drown, Christ has ensured our victory. Our shortcomings and failures are absorbed into *His* victory. Jesus removed the accusatory competitor from the race.

There's nobody else in the pool, Sister!
Hallelujah!

❧

MY PRAYER FOR YOU: Victory in the difficult battles of infertility is what I pray this sweet woman will experience, dear Lord. Her heart is hurting—like lungs which feel as though they'll burst in a demanding swimming event—but You know that and are filled with compassion for her. Please show her when she feels as though You're allowing her to sink that You're really in the process of building her up. Refine her into the beautiful, spiritually athletic woman You have designed her to be: Victorious!

20

The Frail-Hearted Servant

"BRAD," I WHISPERED TENTATIVELY.

"Hmm?"

So he was awake, at least sort of.

"I'm sorry, but I need to talk to you about something."

He didn't ask if it could wait until morning, even though he probably wanted to. It was, after all, time to sleep. I should have brought this conversation up earlier but had tried to discount the need.

"Okay. What did you want to talk about?" he asked willingly but drowsily.

"The procedure we have coming up, the unfinished book, the women I want to minister to who will hate me if I get pregnant." My voice was already beginning to shake. This would obviously be no two-minute delay on my husband's sleep, and I felt badly about that. Brad was silent; he knew me well enough to sense this "talk" needed to start out with listening on his part.

"I really wanted to finish the book on infertility before God gave us a baby. But it's not done yet, and I'm afraid. What if I'm pregnant or we adopt a baby before I get it done? It won't work. It's just… not good."

"Why?" he asked.

"Because the women it's written for will write me off. Nothing I try to share with them will sink in. They'll just feel resentment and abandonment that another Christian with infertility got what she wanted and is now spewing forth advice. They won't accept me as one of them," I explained.

I stared at our bedroom ceiling before continuing. "There's what I call an 'us and them' syndrome. It's like there are two types of married women: the *us* who want children but don't have any and the *them* who do. I'll have changed camps and become one of *them!*" I finally whispered.

Tears fell to my pillow as I struggled for composure. "I want to be a mom but not before the book is done! It wouldn't seem fair. I'll *always* ache with these women in their pain, but they won't be able to know or even believe that."

The counsel I received that night was difficult for me to accept, although it was solid. Brad took me back to the basics:

- Who impressed you to write the book, June? *God did.*
- Who did God choose to write this particular book of encouragement? *Me, but I don't know why.*
- Who will provide us with children if it happens? *God will.*
- When will God give us our children if He does? *At the best time possible, in His perfect timing.*
- Whose book is it? *God's, technically.*

✳ Don't you think God knew in advance how the
timing of all this would work out? *Well, yes.*

Even though I trusted God, I was afraid of becoming one
of *them* and from there feeling ineligible to have a trust relationship with women still in the throes of childlessness. What
I really feared was rejection and the end to a ministry in which
my heart was immersed.

Brad suggested that, like Joshua, I might have to just get my
feet wet with this book as I started to cross the Jordan river.
His spiritual application made me laugh through the tears. He
had no idea it was my *own* example from God's Word in the
chapter I had written long ago about us perhaps having to do
more than just pray in relation to resolving infertility.

Sometimes, God's affirmation was downright *scary!*

⁊

Although it had gone beautifully, the surgical procedure
brought us no closer to becoming parents. I was clearly and
unquestionably *not* pregnant. I cried, of course, for a couple
of minutes before a rushing joy engulfed me. God had *honored*
my petition! He had a better plan for us! I couldn't imagine
what it was, but knew in my heart it was true.

Our pastor at the time learned of the negative pregnancy
test and came over in the hope of encouraging me. He was
devastated by the news, and I loved him for it. Yet we had a
momentary role reversal: I sat on the couch reminding him
of God's sovereignty and how He was working through my
"failed" surgery. Our pastor was finally encouraged by the time
he left.

During the next two days, I had the opportunity to remind my Christian friends who thought God *had* to make our infertility procedure work that He was still on His throne and had a plan. On the third day, the adoption agency called. We were apparently far enough on the list to finally start our home study process! From that point on, we were told, things could happen quickly. I felt we had received clear direction from God and was amazed at how things were coming together.

The call from the adoption agency ushered in a busy, exciting time in which we attended group classes, completed hordes of paperwork, had the required doctors' appointments and fingerprinting done, and met with our gem of a caseworker. We decided against a second surgical procedure. *We were ready to adopt.*

The book was on hold, and there had been no windfall of unexpected cash. I wondered how God was going to provide the money for the adoption fee. I prayed for our baby and his or her birth mother faithfully. Then, suddenly, it seemed, we had only one meeting left to go with our adoption agency. They told us we should have our nursery completely ready. Brad told them it was. Our kindhearted caseworker then asked whether or not we had purchased a car seat, and we nodded in smiling affirmation. The next question, however, caught us both a bit by surprise: "Do you have infant diapers?"

Brad and I both looked like deer in the headlights before I answered we didn't.

"You need to pick some up. You're going to need them," our caseworker said with a sparkle in her eyes.

I caught my breath and asked, "Did a birth mother choose us?"

"I can't tell you. All I can say is that you need to have everything... now."

For not being able to answer my question, she was communicating volumes. As it turned out, we had been chosen by a young lady to be the parents of her unborn baby, and it was both thrilling and humbling. Someone chose *us*, a couple who now lived in an ugly, little four-plex in the middle of nowhere. For all we knew, we could have our adopted baby in a matter of days, or even *hours!* I was dizzy with excitement, and nauseated.

And less than a week later, after five agonizing years of infertility, I numbly found myself staring at my first ever, positive pregnancy test.

꩜

"I'm going to be seeing an infertility specialist next month," an attractive young woman in the Sunday school class we were visiting was saying to another couple. "We're hoping he can help us."

My heart skipped a beat and I felt a rush of love. The Lord provided me with an opportunity to converse with this young lady alone, and she opened up to me about her and her husband's pain-filled infertility. As it turned out, the specialist she was going to go meet with was our own.

"He's *your* doctor?" she asked, stunned.

"Yes," I responded. "I have an infertility problem too."

She glanced at my waistline. "Sure, you do!" she uttered with biting sarcasm before walking away. I stood blinking in confusion and then looked down.

I was six months pregnant and had *forgotten*. I cried all the way home from the worship service, and it was a long commute.

"How can God use *me?*" I wailed miserably. "I'm so stupid! And pregnant! And now I'm an outcast of the infertile society!"

Brad felt sick about it too, but his words were something

along the line of: "God will still use you with them, June. Your burden and love are too great to go unheeded. Be patient and hang in there. God knows what He's doing."

⁂

With a baby officially on the way, I realized the times in the past when I experienced pregnancy-type symptoms were ones in which I had, in fact, been carrying children. I wept for our babies which had died in the womb, even as I wondered in awe what it must be like for those little, precious lives to have never known a moment's heartache or suffering—only life in the presence of Christ in perfection. I marveled that one day we would meet and know each one, whole and healthy.

Brad and I were lovingly kicked out of the agency's adoption process. While everyone was excited for our pregnancy, I found myself with mixed emotions. I stood at the doorway of the nursery and ached at the knowledge a birth mother had chosen us to parent her little son or daughter who would never be sleeping in that room. I felt a wrenching pain and sense of loss over the terminated adoption. I didn't feel I could talk to anyone but God about it. At the same time, I was experiencing deep awe and joy over the life God was forming in my womb, and I was happy for the couple God *really* intended to adopt that baby boy or girl. It was all rather complex for me to process.

⁂

"Isn't this wonderful, June? Now you can finish your book!"

I was fast becoming sorry I had ever asked for prayer from anyone about the writing of this book. I believed my feelings of inadequacy when God first laid it on my heart to write it had been justified, for surely any competent servant of God would have completed it long ago. The nearly finished book now seemed like an elephant in the room. I was both grateful for and uncomfortable with the interest from my friends who had been in prayer about it.

"It's been 90 percent complete for a long time," I would tell them. "I just don't have a feel for how God wants it to finish." *Or what to do with what I wrote before I knew I'd become a mother? Do I change it all? Leave it? Lord God, please help me! I'm so confused.*

While my friends gladly told me I now had a happy ending to my story, I cringed inwardly. How do you explain to a person who's never experienced infertility that you'd rather face a firing squad than tell "my happy story" to a woman aching for her own baby?

I humbly shared with them how difficult it is to hear other people's success stories when you don't have the baby you long for. "The book's focus has to remain on *God's truths*. God is the only One who can offer meaningful hope in this painful walk!"

❧

I don't know what You want, Lord. What's the final chapter to be? Am I to be writing? Giving up? What? My questions were met with complete silence. Did that mean I was to be waiting?

In my uncertainty, I made the decision to hold onto the things I was certain *of:* all the truths and encouragements God had previously and mercifully shared with me. He had a plan, and it was on time.

❧

That illusive chapter, I later learned, would be about a Father's love. It was something I had to experience, however, before it could be written.

The pregnancy went smoothly, and Brad and I were blessed with a daughter. We named her Tina. I had no post-partum depression and felt wonderful. We were grateful for the miracle God had done. Yet to my relief, I felt no different from the women I knew who were still weeping for a child, and they could sense that. God, in His love and graciousness, enabled me to keep ministering. It was *my* phone which rang when someone with infertility needed a friend to talk to. To this day, I am humbled and grateful for that.

After Tina was born, I seemed to conceive almost easily, but suffered more miscarriages. We became an official "secondary infertility" couple. Then God gave us Samuel, the result of an amazing, second successful pregnancy. One of my friends started calling me Lucky Dog June.

Unknown to me, with Sam's arrival the stage was set for the final chapter. And God knew *exactly* how He wanted it. It was to be His declaration of unconditional, unfathomable love.

And I'm thankful I didn't know in advance His plan.

MY PRAYER FOR YOU: Father God, if this dear reader, who was in Your mind and heart the day You so clearly instructed me to write this book, has been focusing on my story as opposed to You, I ask You to please change that at this moment. May I disappear behind the cross of Christ and Your beauty, and may she see with stunning clarity Your breathtaking love for her. May she read on and be overwhelmed by the goodness of You. Amen.

21

A Father's Love

"WELL, JUNE, are you ready for tomorrow?"

The man asking the question looked strangely frail and superhuman at the same time. Lines of fatigue etched his face, yet his hospital garb and paper-covered shoes intimidated me.

"Yes," came my quiet, firm reply.

It was late at night, but I'd come to learn it never seemed to matter at the pediatric intensive care unit. No matter the hour, people were always up and about.

I wondered how well rested the surgeon would be for what was to be required of him in a matter of hours. I looked at his hands and prayed they would be steady. His reputation was tremendous; there was some degree of comfort in that.

Looking suddenly like a father, the surgeon walked to the sterile hospital bed I was now accustomed to. He gazed at Samuel. At not quite seven weeks of age, Sam didn't take up too much space. The man's expression momentarily softened before he seemed to steel himself and turn back to me with piercing eyes.

"Do you have any questions about the surgery?"

I shook my head. "No. His doctors have been very clear and patient in explaining to us what will take place."

There was a slight pause before his next question. "Then, although we are not anticipating any problems, you *do* understand Sam could die either during surgery or from complications resulting from it?"

"Yes," I answered as the undeniable presence of God again encompassed me. "We know there's that chance. But we also know he will die for a certainty if he *doesn't* have surgery."

The man nodded. "Very good; tomorrow, then." He shook my hand and left.

Yes, tomorrow. A big day.

I was tired and thought I should try to get at least a little sleep, but I knew Brad was planning on another long trip to the hospital that night. Besides, I enjoyed looking at Sam, and it wouldn't hurt to feast my eyes on this miracle baby a while longer.

⁂

Sam's arrival into the world went smoothly. Except for being more than three weeks early and having a bout with jaundice, he was coming on strong. We were grateful to have another child—another *healthy* child at that. Tina was excited at the miracle of her brother, and it was an indescribably happy time in our lives.

Sam's initial checkups were fine; he was growing and slowly gaining weight. However, at a five-week follow-up his pediatrician was uncomfortable with his breathing patterns. One mild concern led to another before she scheduled an appointment for Sam with a pediatric Cardiologist.

"His heart is probably just fine," she said earnestly after conducting an ultrasound on it. "But I just want to make sure." I appreciated her concern. Two of her colleagues had openly scoffed at her unease when she'd called them in for additional opinions.

While driving Sam to the appointment with the heart specialist the following morning, I was listening to the local Christian radio station. They played one of my favorite songs: "It Is Well with My Soul." It was an instrumental version in my low voice range, so I sang while driving down the highway, affected, as always, by the song's powerful message of assurance in God's faithfulness even in suffering. Afterward, the announcer said, "I wasn't planning on playing that song, but suddenly felt someone was going to sustain a blow today and thought it might help them, somehow."

Oh, Lord! I remember praying, *whoever that may be, help them to remember this song and be strengthened by it!*

༈

Two hours later, I knew Sam was in trouble. The cardiologist explained that our "healthy little boy" had a birth defect causing over a 90 percent blockage in his aorta, which supplies blood to the lower extremities. His blood pressure was through the roof. In summary, Sam was a ticking time bomb ready to go off at any moment. He needed major heart surgery *immediately*.

I didn't break down until I phoned Brad at work. A staff nurse then walked Sam and me across the street to the hospital. His condition was so critical we bypassed registration completely. "Don't worry about admittance formalities," the doctors said. "Paperwork is not a concern right now."

I sat down in tears and started to shake. My control was slipping, and I prayed for strength. Suddenly, I remembered the song on the radio:

When peace like a river attendeth my way
When sorrows like sea billows roll
Whatever my lot, Thou hast taught me to say,
It is well, it is well with my soul.

Oh, God! I cried silently, *You played that song on the radio for me? For me!*

God immediately brought to my mind the words from our pastor's sermon just *three days earlier.* He and his family were facing a crisis and God had clearly impressed upon them this crisis was *in the plan.* The plan God had set down before the creation of the world.

The perfect plan of God which was unfolding precisely on schedule.

It became instantly clear why little Sam and I were in the intensive care unit. It was "in the plan." We were right on schedule. Then and there, I turned my fears and questions over to God and committed myself to "bloom where I was planted."

Sam's heart responded immediately to the medication they gave him, and his dangerously high blood pressure dropped significantly. The cardiologist looked less strained.

"Good boy, Sam!" he said before adding: "Now we might be able to *schedule* his surgery and get the surgeon I want!"

I found myself having to think about and absorb a great deal of information in a short amount of time. My thoughts turned towards Tina. I was grateful God had led me to leave her with Paige for this particular doctor's appointment. I wondered if she was having fun; I also wondered if she were going to lose her little brother.

How I longed to have Brad at my side! I wondered what he must be feeling as he made his way from work into the city.

❧

"This blood test we're taking here is to test for RSV. It's a pneumonia virus which is running rampant through the county and can be fatal to infants." The nurse was repeating what the cardiologist had already told me, but I didn't mind. It gave me a chance to see how well I comprehended things the first time around.

Sam was screaming in loud protest while they drew his blood. *You've had so many pokes already, and the worst is yet to come,* I thought in anguish. I continued to pray silently and fervently on his behalf.

"We're checking any little ones going into surgery just as a precaution. Anesthesia on a baby causes some collapsing of the lungs. The lungs recover from it. But pneumonia causes the same thing and surgery *plus* RSV would be, well, too much," she finished lamely.

"As in totally collapsed lungs?" I asked.

"Right," she continued, business-like again. "But it's obvious that Sam doesn't have the virus. Our good, little boy doesn't even have a sniffle." The nurse's voice had resumed to what I determined to be a natural tenderness, reminding me of one of our family members. *Oh, no!* It occurred to me. *They'll need to know what's going on!*

"Well, Sam," I gently breathed. "We need to fix your poor little heart, but at least you don't have RSV. See, Honey? Things really *could* be worse." He was still crying as I stroked his tiny, fuzzy head.

⁊⁊

The nurse's face was pale, even though her voice was composed. "Sam has tested RSV positive, Mrs. Strickler. You will be required to suit up to be with him. The doctor is on his way over."

I saw tears building up in her eyes before she turned away to other duties.

⁊⁊

The doctor didn't come alone. There were several: cardiologists and infectious disease specialists, an ICU physician, and I'm not really sure what all else. I had believed I was becoming better at rolling with the punches, but this one nearly downed me.

"We've got to have a new game plan." One of the cardiologists was saying. "This is a bad turn of events. We *cannot* perform surgery until the baby works through the pneumonia; unless his heart begins to go and then, of course, we'll have no choice but to take him in as is."

I was no medical genius, but even I knew a five-week old baby with a bad heart was not going to flourish with pneumonia.

⁊⁊

An old enemy came to call. I could actually feel an evil presence close behind me on my right side; it literally raised the hair on the back of my neck.

Ask God "why?"

Get angry! who wouldn't in your place?

246

Curse God! He could have prevented this!

Tears welled up in my eyes and spilled over. I clutched the railing to Sam's hospital bed with my sweaty, rubber-gloved hands. The gloves, gown, and mask I was required to wear seemed to suffocate me. I hated them. I hated all of this.

I won't! I argued silently and stubbornly in response to the enemy's temptations. *God is all I have left to cling to! Leave me, Satan! I'm claiming Romans 8:28. I know that God causes all things to work together for good to those who love God, to those who are called according to His purpose, and I will not deny God now!*

※

I watched Sam sleep fitfully and thought about the surgeon's visit to our room and his words. The RSV was at last behind us. Sam had barely survived. We could again touch our child with ungloved hands. Now all we had to contend with were the temperamental clamps and cords for his monitoring equipment, and they no longer caused me distress.

Yes, I realized. *I'm ready for the surgery tomorrow.*

It was incredible to me Sam was alive and strong enough for the operation. There had been a stretch when nobody would have placed odds on his making it through the pneumonia. It was indeed a miracle. Where the thought of major heart surgery had at first frightened us, it was now an answer to prayer and something we were immensely thankful for.

Several amazing things had happened in the previous two weeks. God had sustained us by the prayers of family, friends, and multiple strangers (some worldwide) who had learned of Sam's plight. God had turned Sam's listing from ICU/critical condition to ICU/fair condition in less than a two-hour period, to the utter amazement of the physicians and nurses. God had enabled me to share the reason for our strength through the darkest hours to countless hospital personnel and staff who questioned us about it. God caused a friend's toddler to cough on and off through Sam's most dangerous night, keeping this friend awake and looking through her living room window at the very hospital she knew Sam was in. She cared for her toddler and prayed for Sam all night. (Notably, this friend's same child was perfectly fine and cough-free before and after that specific time of prayer when Sam was going under.) God also enabled us to place two Bibles in a non-Christian home.

We were exhausted and still concerned for Sam but feeling a bit exhilarated as well. He was alive! He was going to have his needed surgery! The doctors were now optimistic, almost gloating. I was actually feeling somewhere between contented and elated. God's plan was beginning to appear Sam would be going *home* with us! It seemed like a thousand years had passed. Walking out the front door of the hospital with our baby in my arms would be the strangest feeling I could imagine.

Despite the strain he'd been under, I could tell Brad's faith was intact as he entered Sam's room. We had been assisted by friends and family members and my sister, at great personal sacrifice to herself and family, was staying at our home to help with communications, home management, and Tina. Brad had made the hour-long drive into the hospital after Tina had gone to bed. We talked about the next day's events and traded "health and hospital" news for "Tina, home-front, and telephone message" news. Brad was relieved to learn everything was still on for surgery in the morning.

"I just want them to fix Sam's heart so we can take him home," he said wearily. "He's been through too much as it is."

As we talked softly amid the beeps and blips of the monitoring equipment, I learned a good friend of ours, who was involved in an organization which taught non-biblical beliefs about God and Jesus Christ, asked Brad if we would like him and a leader from his group to come and pray over Sam before surgery. I was so touched by that friend's love and concern for our son, and so *saddened* and *frustrated* at his lost spiritual state when he thought he was on the "inside track" with God. It had always made sharing with him the good news of freedom in Christ difficult.

"Do you think he'll ever come to know the true Christ, Brad? It seems impossible he will."

Brad responded it *was* possible before saying, "Maybe *this* is what God will use to draw John to a saving knowledge of Jesus Christ."

After Brad left, I sat awhile longer in the room. Since God had enabled me to resist dwelling on certain fears and discouraging facts through this time of trial, I was surprised when my thoughts kept returning to what the surgeon had asked me earlier.

"You do understand Sam could die?"

Almost from the *start* I had known he could die. And just days earlier, when the pneumonia was at its peak, I watched Sam struggling as he grew weaker and weaker. I was there when the doctors looked at me with dull eyes and the nurses and respiratory therapists tried to hide their own fears from me. Oh, *I knew*. Our primary physician had taught me how to read Sam's chest X-rays and had given me free access to the X-ray reading room any time I wanted. I had *seen* his latest X-rays when I felt the flame of life was flickering. I'd stood in numb horror as I surveyed the undeniable evidence in black and white. Both lungs were almost *completely* collapsed.

I *had* faced the reality Sam might never come home with us. Yet, through it all, my aching heart had repeatedly turned to God.

I trust You to do what's best, dear Lord. But please, give me the strength to honor You through this.

Sam is Yours and always has been. Please spare his life if that is what's best for the cause of Christ.

Lord, God, I know this is working for good. Yet I beg You to make it a lot of good. This is too awful, too hard to have just a little good come of it!

God and His Word had sustained me and sent perplexed non-Christian hospital workers to me with questions about my unwavering love for God. He even used us as a couple to build up the faith of some of our Christian friends. So why the worry *now?*

But Brad's statement and the surgeon's began playing a duet in my exhausted mind.

You do understand that Sam could die?

Maybe this is what God will use to draw John.

Could it still be we weren't out of the woods, I wondered? Was it yet possible God's plan was for us to lose our son and Tina to lose her new, little brother?

Of *course*, it was possible! My mind shouted. Wasn't *I* the one who didn't want others to try and put God in a box? Should *we* somehow be immune to the pain of loss the couple in the room next door just experienced with *their* newborn son? Was *our* child somehow more important than anyone *else's?*

No! God was *God*. He could do whatever He deemed best. And it might *be* His plan to call Sam home to Himself, even yet!

As I sat in the semi-dark room, I struggled to think lovingly and openly about those facts. I contemplated the possible trade-off between the life of our innocent baby and the spiritual salvation of our friend. I weighed them carefully in my mind, as I strove to see what I thought may be God's possible logic in this trial. In my humanness, it suddenly seemed ridiculous, horrid, and unfathomable to me.

"God!" I cried in my heart. *"John's a pretty good guy and You know how much we love him! But You wouldn't use Sam's death to save him, would you? It's not an equal tradeoff. Even at his best, I'm not sure John's worth that; the cost would be far, far, too great!"*

The moment I came to grips with my honest assessment, God's response instantly breathed its way through my being:

> *I gave My Son. He was perfect and blameless. Was that an equal trade-off? The Son of God for the sinful human race?*

So great was the confrontation, I was unable to breathe for a moment. *Oh, God, no!* I agonized silently. *None of us were worth that cost!*

I was touched—and horrified—but not yet through with my wrestling. Tears streamed down my face, and so intense were my feelings, this time I spoke out loud. Like Abraham pleading with God before the destruction of Sodom and Gomorrah (see Genesis 18:16-33), I felt I was trying to sway the iron will of God.

If You must take Sam, please bring more people to salvation through it than just John. Save hundreds... thousands! Oh, God! One soul is not worth the life of our baby!

Then God planted these words in my mind:

I loved you enough. Had you been the only sinner on the face of the earth, I still would have given My Son. I would have followed through with salvation's plan, for even one.

I had always been taught that God would have sent His Son for just one. However, for the first time in my life, that truth left me trembling. In the subdued lighting of the hospital room, I appreciated my salvation as I had never been able to do before. A true glimpse of the Father's love left me incapable of all but the deepest fear and awe for what He had done for a sinful human race.

At the greatest cost imaginable, He gave His Son for me, and for you.

Oh, God, I whispered brokenly. *I've never, never thanked You enough!*

❧

The surgery went very well. I was full of joy and a new humbleness. There was much rejoicing in the home ranks and elsewhere as the news spread to those who had stood by us in prayer. I was so happy and relieved, at first I failed to notice I had a fever.

❧

"Did I wish you a happy birthday?" Brad asked. "I honestly can't remember."

I was huddled in a room at the Ronald McDonald House where I would shower and occasionally catch a little sleep. It was Brad at the hospital now, updating me. Sam's heart surgery had been on Monday. Tuesday I was sick and feverish after being by him in his recovery. Sam had been losing more fluids than the normal drainage. The doctors were concerned they might have to operate again to locate and repair the problem. In the meantime, we discovered I had come down with a variety of stomach flu and could pose an additional danger to the baby by staying with him. So it was that Wednesday found me on the phone with Brad.

"How are you feeling, June?"

"I'm better, but still a bit feverish. It's Sam I want to know about. What are his fluids doing? How did things go last night?"

My heart froze as I learned Sam was going into surgery again, right away.

"I'll be down to the hospital in a few minutes," I said.

"June," Brad interposed. "There's nothing you can do and the flu is the last thing Sam needs. You should stay where you are and try to rest and get well. I'll keep you posted as soon as I know something."

I began to sob. "What kind of a mother would lie in bed while her baby is having surgery, Brad? I can't do that. I've *got* to be there!"

I was torn. How I wanted to be there for our son—and myself. But I didn't want to expose him to the flu. It was then I did what I knew to be right, although I hated it with all my being: I went back to bed.

It was the longest, most awful day I had ever experienced. I tried sleeping and praying, all to no avail. God's presence was still indescribably real to me, but I felt as though He was blocking me from Sam in every way possible. It took a valiant and determined effort for me to not ask God, *Why?*

Brad finally called. The surgery had been long and difficult. The surgeon was frustrated; he hadn't been able to make the repair the way he wanted, but it *was* done. Sam should be fine. He was coming out of his anesthesia, and Brad would keep me posted.

I just felt like crying.

God! I want to be by his side. I know there's nothing I can do, but he's my son! I hate this awful separation when he needs me!

There was only silence which seemed to stretch on endlessly.

After what felt like an eternity, Brad again called, and he sounded terrible. Sam was in obvious pain, he told me. He was thrashing and being restrained. He kept gagging on his respirator tube. Medications didn't seem to be helping.

"It's awful, June. I just can't stand to see him suffer like this."

After the call, I hit my knees in prayer.

God, I love You but hate what is happening to Sam! Please free him from his pain. I beg You! The pneumonia, heart problems, and fear of losing him were all hard, but God, I can't stand the thought of him in such pain. Please take it away! Oh, God, please take it away now!

It seemed I could accept everything but that little one in such pain. I wept, cried, and begged. At last, I uttered my heart's desire:

Lord, please relieve Sam's pain or just hurry and take him home to be with You!

It was suddenly like Sunday night again when God's Spirit had planted words in my mind about the Father's love.

He could have called ten thousand angels.

This phrase from an old hymn ran through my mind. I suddenly thought of God and *His* Son.

While Christ was on the cross becoming sin for us, He was

separated from His Father; God had to turn His back on His only Son at the most difficult time in Jesus' ministry. And God had *known* from the start it would be that way! Unlike God, I didn't have to hear my son cry out, *"Why have You forsaken me?"*

❀

Until that very moment, I'd never really grasped the immense *pain* God felt when He "so loved the world that He gave His only begotten Son." Unlike God, I would have done anything in my power to reach down and remove my son from his pain.

God had the power, and, I might add, every *right* to stop the proceedings on Calvary's cross—and His only Son's pain and anguish. Yet He didn't. He *didn't!* Because of us, whose sin *caused* His pain!

❀

Soon after my impassioned prayer, Sam was resting comfortably. We ended up taking him home with us, weighing less than he did at birth but healthy, inside and out. Christ's agony on the cross of Calvary, I must note, was not shortened. God loved humanity enough to suffer the ultimate pain and pay the ultimate price:

> *For God **so loved** the world, that He gave His only*
> *begotten Son, that whoever believes in Him*
> *should not perish, but have eternal life.*
> *John 3:16*

Can you imagine such a love? Perhaps not. But it's a love we can *trust in*.

It's breathtaking hope.

❧

Are you one of Christ's? Are you a Christian as God describes in the Bible (as opposed to how our culture does)? If so, when was the last time you shed tears of gratitude for the immeasurable gift of salvation God gave to you? How long has it been since you said, *Thank You* with every ounce of your being to your Creator God and Savior? To the Spirit who opened your eyes and heart, drawing you into repentance and God's family?

I sweetly encourage you to *keep seeking* God for a child, even as I must ask: Have you recently been moved to tears of thankfulness for the child He *already* gave you? Have you wept on behalf of the child of God Himself, who—being fully God and fully man—died in the prime of life for our sins? The Messiah King who rose from the grave three days later and now intercedes on your behalf, who loves you more than we can ever comprehend?

If it's been awhile, it's time, my sister. It's time *now*.

❧

This book addresses every issue as if you are one of Christ's followers, yet I recognize you may never have accepted God's gift of forgiveness and salvation through His Son, Jesus Christ. Perhaps you haven't understood before this moment how much God loves you and desires to have intimate fellowship with you. If such is the case, you can become a part of God's family today, *right now,* by crying out to God your desire to be His. Surely you feel the weight of your sin and long to be rid of it and experience God's gracious forgiveness. Tell Him that. Ask Him for forgiveness and to adopt you through Jesus Christ, whom you want to serve and give your life to, no matter who may persecute you, no matter what further tests, trials, and heartaches may come your way. If you're willing, tell Him that.

It's time, my dear friend. It's time *now*.

※

He who did not spare His own Son, but delivered Him up for us all, how will He not also with Him freely give us all things? Who will bring a charge against God's elect? God is the one who justifies; who is the one who condemns? Christ Jesus is He who died, yes, rather who was raised, who is at the right hand of God, who also intercedes for us.

Who shall separate us from the love of Christ? Shall tribulation, or distress, or persecution, or famine, or nakedness, or peril, or sword? Just as it is written, 'For thy sake we are being put to death all day long; we were considered as sheep to be slaughtered.' But in all these things we overwhelmingly conquer through Him who loved us.

For I am convinced that neither death, nor life, nor angels, nor principalities, nor things present, nor things to come, nor powers, nor height, nor depth, nor any other created thing, shall be able to separate us from the love of God which is in Christ Jesus our Lord. (Romans 8:32-39)

As miserable as infertility is, it cannot separate those of us who are in Christ Jesus from the Father's love. *Nothing can.* The Father's love remains powerful and pure no matter what we face or how we choose to question or view it.

❧

In times when all seems hopeless, we're often brought to the basics. For the child of God, that basic is to rest in and rediscover His unfathomable, perfect love. It's breathtaking today. And tomorrow. And into eternity.

I love you even if we've never met. And I pray you will become a joyful mother, a passionate lover of the Lord Jesus Christ, and an encouragement and light to all whose lives you touch.

This book has never been about me. It's about you and the God who loves you with beauty and power. And when the last word here has been read, the story—of God's merciful pursuit of intimacy with you—will continue. Be in awe of Him, cherished daughter of the King, and let Him write His story in you.

> Now unto Him who is able to keep you from stumbling, and to make you stand in the presence of His glory blameless with great joy, to the only God our Savior, through Jesus Christ our Lord, be glory, majesty, dominion and authority, before all time and now and forever. Amen. (Jude 24-25)

ACKNOWLEDGMENTS

There would have been no such thing as a meaningful book entitled *Breathtaking Hope in the Furnace of Infertility* were it not for the treasure trove of individuals God used through the ages to faithfully sacrifice, translate, share, and joyfully display the glory of His person and His word. Their names are on an eternal list, kept and revered in heaven—waiting for the day to be showcased before the whole of creation. Well done good and faithful servants.

Brad, thank you for being my husband-friend and helping me to finish well with this book. You're the best encourager an encourager could have, and I love you.

If I were to give an Endurance Award to those who've loved and stood by me on this project (like *forever*), it would certainly to go to you, Becky Gibbons and Harriett Donovan. Thank you, friends. Also, thank you my giving first round draft reviewers: Danica Middleton, Becky Guinn, and Candace Tucker. My eternal thanks also rise to God for Sue Hepner, a first round book reviewer and true, kindred spirit whose faith in Jesus Christ has since become sight. To her beloved husband and family, thank you. You helped to make Sue the special person that she was, and her legacy continues in many ways—including the completion of this book she so prayer-fully and sweetly petitioned God about.

I'm also honored to publicly thank you, my faithful second round book reviewers: Gi Gi Horrell, Anna Stewart, Deborah Clendon, Diana Mayhugh, and Beryl Forney. You sharpened my writing and thinking through the final drafting process and gave me courage to stay the course. I was afraid you'd be mean, but you weren't!

To the team of organizers, leaders, writers, presenters, and par-ticipants of the annual Colorado Christian Writers Conference, thank you. God used you greatly to get this, *His* message of breathtaking hope, to women longing for motherhood.

Thank you, also, Geoffrey Stone. You were highly recom-mended to me as a professional editor and surpassed my hope-ful expectations. Your tremendous skill, insight, and patience combined to make delicate improvements to the quality of this book. And, your, comma, reduction, plan, will, no, doubt, bless, my, readers!

Erik Peterson, your professional layout of the book's interior and cover design are deeply appreciated. Thank you for creat-ing a cover which reflects the power and hope available to us through the breathtaking God of creation. You knocked it out of the ball park!

ABOUT THE AUTHOR

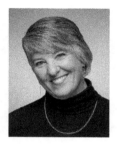

June Strickler is a writer, blogger, public speaker, and Founding Director of Encouragement That Lasts, a 501(c)(3) nonprofit corporation. She is a member of the Christian Independent Publishers Association (CIPA) and an actively volunteers. Her experience in the legal field, county administration, local and global church ministries, crisis intervention, and the home provide a basis for her refreshing and unique diversity. June thrills in proclaiming God's truths and how His flagrant grace and intimacy is available to everyone. Sign up to receive June's blogs and receive encouragement which transcends the cultural norm at:

WWW.ENCOURAGEMENTTHATLASTS.ORG

Encouragement THAT LASTS

Join the growing list of those receiving
Encouragement That Lasts blogs and releases at:

WWW.ENCOURAGEMENTTHATLASTS.ORG

CPSIA information can be obtained
at www.ICGtesting.com
Printed in the USA
BVHW062055250221
601128BV00014B/1477